Would you believe it, doctor?

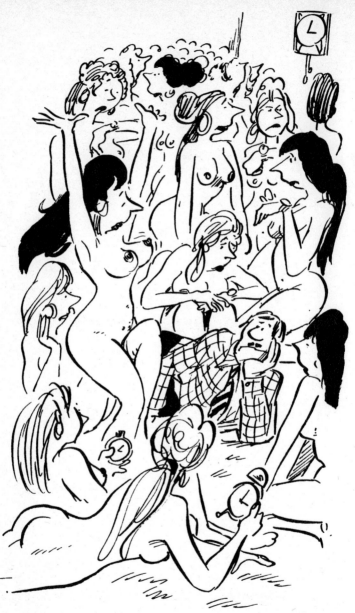

Young men think about sex once every 15 minutes

Would you believe it, doctor?

DICK AND ROSE GIRLING
JOHN AND JACKIE RUNECKLES
RICK AND DEIDRE SANDERS

Arthur Barker Limited
A subsidiary of Weidenfeld (Publishers) Limited

Arthur Barker Limited
11 St John's Hill London SW11

ISBN 0 213 16561 9

Photosetting by
TRI-AM Photoset Ltd.
Bridge Foot, Warrington

Printed and bound in Great Britain by
Morrison & Gibb Ltd., London and Edinburgh

Illustrated by Bill Tidy

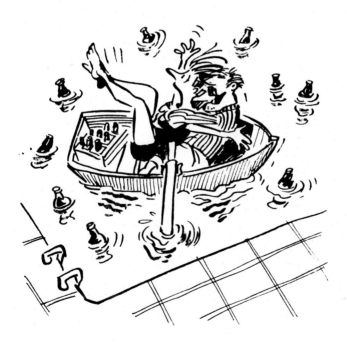

Owl broth was used in Yorkshire as a remedy against whooping cough.

During the early years of her reign, Queen Victoria employed an official bearing the title Her Majesty's Bug Destroyer.

A study in Toronto in 1963 showed that people who drove more than 12,000 miles a year were twice as likely to develop cancer as those who stayed nearer home.

In 1960 R. F. Leggett and T. D. Northwood carried out an investigation to determine whether or not the noise at cocktail parties might be a health hazard to diplomats. They concluded that the maximum babble level was not quite high enough to cause permanent deafness.

Among the casualties treated at Farnborough Hospital, Kent, in 1965 was a patient who had been injured by an exploding pudding.

Physicians in Henry VIII's day had an adequate grasp of the principles of contagion, but were a trifle weak on the mechanics. The king's venereal disease was put down to Cardinal Wolsey and the fact that he had been whispering in his master's ear.

Staff at a nursing home were puzzled when elderly men urinated every time the local lifeboat was launched. It turned out that the electronic emptying devices connected to the patients' partially paralysed bladders operated on the same wavelength as the lifeboat's radio.

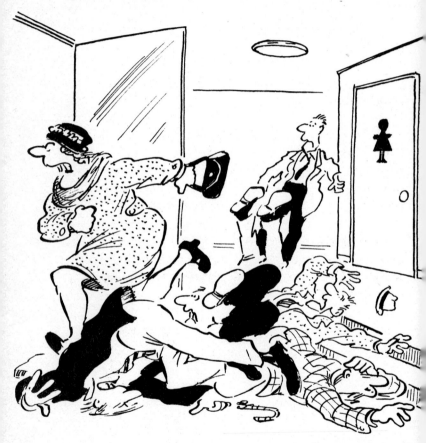

Research has shown that a woman can use a public lavatory and be out in the street again in 45 seconds.

Favourite discussion topics among teenage boys are, in preference order, drugs, boy-girl relationships, vd, alcohol, contraception, marriage and human reproduction. Girls favour vd, boy-girl relationships, child-parent relationships, marriage, drugs, child-care and cancer.

The average slipped disc costs its Western owner £2 a day.

Your skin is a twentieth of an inch thick and weighs about six pounds.

A Californian burial-at-sea club (the Neptune Club, 'offering competitive rates') guarantees to cast your ashes from a real Grecian urn, outside the three mile limit, while the ship's captain reads a choice of a poem by Tennyson or the 107th psalm.

Choristers in the Vatican owe a lasting debt of gratitude to Pope Leo xiii for a liberal ruling in the 1890s. He discontinued the practice of having them castrated.

People who keep budgies and canaries are more than usually susceptible to diseases of the heart valve.

Your brain is 85 per cent water.

The Public Health Act of 1842 made it an offence to deposit excrement on the highway.

Gum-chewing is a common cause of flatulence.

Dr Paul Niehans, famous for his work on cell therapy treatments, shocked Zurich's polite citizens by appearing at a fancy dress party disguised as a rectal thermometer.

Prime Minister Gladstone, depicted vigorously brandishing an axe, appeared on a nineteenth-century advertisement proclaiming: 'Can you afford to die? Can you afford to drag on a miserable existence? Can you afford to pay doctor's bills? When all disorders of the Nervous System, Impaired Vitality and Defective Organic Action can be speedily, effectually and permanently cured by wearing the Electropathic (Battery) Belt.'

A Texan criminal successfully removed the telltale pattern of his fingerprints. He was subsequently identified by his smooth fingertips and ten small oval graft scars on his chest.

More colds develop on Monday than any other day of the week.

Babies have tastebuds all over the insides of their mouths, but by the time they reach adulthood only those on the tongue are left.

It was once fashionable to have all the teeth pulled, in the belief that they could poison the rest of the body.

Wounded soldiers in the Kaiser's army were punished if they did not lie to attention in their hospital beds, with arms stiffly outstretched over the blankets.

10

St Appollonia qualified for the patron sainthood of toothache by having her teeth knocked out by an anti-Christian mob at Alexandria in AD 249. St Erasmus of Elmo earned patronage of the abdomen by having his guts drawn out by a windlass in AD 303. St Lawrence was assigned to the back as a reward for his request, uttered while being roasted on a gridiron in AD 258, to be turned over as his back was now quite done. St Lucy, martyred in AD 304, was given custody of eyes, but was later confused with St Triduana of Scotland who, when her eyes were admired by a pagan lover, plucked them out and presented them to him on a skewer. The patron saint of piles was the sixth century Irishman St Fiacre.

The world constipation record is 102 days.

Philitas of Cos, the Greek grammarian and poet, was said by Atheneus in 300 BC to be so small and thin that he wore lead balls fastened to his shoes to stop him being blown over in high winds.

Spanish husbands commonly take to their beds with abdominal pains when their wives go into labour.

Seventy-six British people die of bronchitis every day. Of these, no more than three will be non-smokers from country districts.

French Academician Henrion insisted that man has been steadily shrinking in stature. To illustrate his thesis, in 1718, he calculated that Adam had stood 123 ft 9 in tall, and Eve 118 ft. He placed in descending order Noah, at 100 ft; Abraham, 80 ft; Moses, 30 ft; Hercules, 10 ft and Alexander the (not very) Great, 6 ft.

Bed bugs travel from room to room in search of victims.

Major advances in our understanding of the digestive system were made in the 1830s by a US Army doctor, William Beaumont, with the help of a French-Canadian trapper named Alexis St Martin. The trapper's stomach had been blasted away in a shooting accident some years before, leaving him with a hole permanently open to the air. Beaumont used this hole in a series of experiments to observe the passage of food and drink through the stomach. He also lowered pieces of food through the cavity on lengths of string, periodically withdrawing them to see how digestion was progressing.

Gamekeeper's Thumb is an injury to which skiers are particularly prone.

The fashion for dwarfs in Italy was pursued to such lengths that parents anointed their children with bat-grease, vole-grease, shrew-grease and tiny-creature-grease in general to inhibit normal growth.

Marshal Blucher, one of Wellington's allies at Waterloo, lived in fear that he would one day give birth to an elephant.

Among the 60,000 tablets, 220 ampoules and 5 litres of liquid medicine surrendered during the opening 4 days of a 'return unwanted medicines' campaign in Oxfordshire in 1974 were 8 thalidomide tablets, enough potassium cyanide and arsenic to kill more than 2000 people, and a 50-year-old bottle of worm syrup.

Castration is the only foolproof way to prevent baldness.

In 1830 a half-hundredweight tumour was cut from a Chinaman who had travelled all the way to London for his operation, which was performed before an audience of 680 people. The patient's death was said to have nothing to do with the fact that the operation took two hours and was done without anaesthetic. The deciding factor was the foulness of the air poisoned by so many onlookers.

Romans warded off heart attacks by sucking milk from the breasts of slaves and eating dog excrement.

Fifty million of your cells will have died while you have been reading this sentence.

A British survey in 1972 revealed that 1639 people had been infected with gonorrhoea from a single source.

Gaspare Tagliacozzi in the sixteenth century tried to transplant noses, lips and ears.

Pliny the Elder's corn cure required the sufferer to keep an eye on the stars while someone poured oil on to the hinge of a door.

Eau de Cologne was invented as a protection against plague.

Casanova's favoured contraceptive devices included a sheath made from sheep's intestine, half a lemon used as a Dutch cap, and 2 oz gold balls, also for use by his partners.

James Paget, discoverer of Paget's disease of the nipple and, for a while, Queen Victoria's Sergeant Surgeon, ended his presidential address to the Pathological Society of London with a sentence of 78 consecutive monosyllables.

The first recorded operation to remove an ovarian cyst was performed in Danville, Kentucky, by Ephraim McDowell in 1809. Lacking anaesthesia, the patient, a Mrs Crawford, sustained herself by singing hymns.

In 1968 the US Government paid a dollar each for 24,000 bottles of physiological sodium chloride – a special saline solution for use in hospital laboratories. The bottles contained ordinary seawater.

Science has found an infallible cure for insomnia. All you need is a series of momentary electric shocks, delivered at a steady rhythm and synchronised with four flashing lights placed before your eyes, which must be glued open. If shocks and lights are then both synchronised with the beat of loud jazz music, you will be asleep within minutes. It's guaranteed.

A modern estimate puts Goethe's IQ at 210; Voltaire and Newton at 190; Galileo 185; Leonardo and Descartes 180; Lincoln 150; Napoleon 145; Washington 140 and Drake and General Grant 130.

Research has shown that people who claim to be able to wake up at a particular hour actually wake repeatedly until the stipulated time is reached.

Ayrshire coalminers were indignant when their first aid examination papers included a number of questions about emergencies in childbirth.

14

Dr Koch's *Glyoxylide* was supposed to cure cancer and tuberculosis, and made its inventor more than $100,000 a year. In 1943 it was chemically analysed as 'indistinguishable from distilled water'.

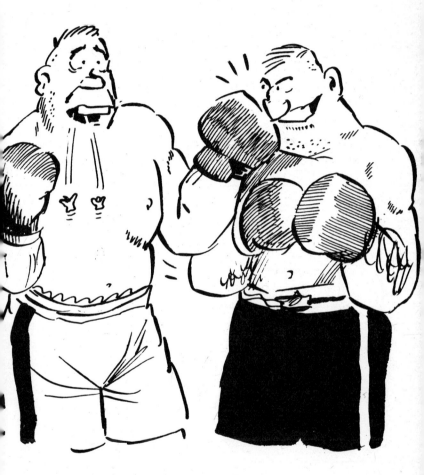

Teeth can be transplanted, but they tend to fall out after a year or two.

London's Marylebone Council objected to the Anti Vivisection League's application to use premises in Harley Street on the grounds that such a use would be out of keeping with the character of the area.

A nurse dismissed from a Birmingham hospital for spitting in front of the matron claimed she was courteously disposing of her chewing gum before addressing her superior.

Extroverts sleep better than introverts.

A Scottish woman avoided the shame of having to reveal that her husband was in hospital with TB by telling the neighbours that he was in prison.

The average woman has a 28-inch waist. The average man's arm is 28 inches long.

Laboratory tests have shown that some aphrodisiac creams on sale in sex supermarkets are chemically similar to rheumatism ointment, though less concentrated.

When Australian Aborigines, accustomed to posing for tourists' cameras, were invited to take advantage of a free radiography service in the sixties, they demanded modelling fees before they would stand in front of the X-ray machines.

Shock makes your blood go sticky.

A Parisienne student was filmed having the Eiffel Tower tattooed on her bottom. The skin was later detached and sold to a collector.

Doctors in China were so revered that it was thought sufficient for patients just to swallow their written prescriptions.

According to civil servant Mr B. E. Reilly, Jack The Ripper was Dr Merchant, a Brixton GP.

Hand preference was almost equally divided among primitive men. It was not until the Bronze Age that people became predominantly right-handed. Now, less than 10 per cent are left-handed.

Few British women reach the age of 40 without a bunion.

Most normal men breath mainly through one nostril for three hours, and mainly through the other for the next three.

In eighteenth-century Germany it was thought that the best cure for mental illness was terror. A favourite method was to tie patients to a rope, raise them to a great height and then plunge them into a dark cellar or, better still, a pit full of snakes.

A Munich doctor selling 'anti-baby marmalade' was arrested when it was discovered that his product consisted mainly of pea-paste.

British blood is growing hotter. According to the Polish daily *Expres Posnanski* in 1968: 'Because of the increased sexuality of the Anglo-Saxons, it was proved possible to exceed our planned output of mistletoe.'

The bark of the pomegranate tree cures diarrhoea and kills tapeworms.

17

Favourite contraceptives among Egyptian women at the time of the pharaohs were elephant and crocodile dung pessaries, and a pint of honey used intra-vaginally.

Doctors in Florida have found that patients undergoing certain operations bleed twice as freely when the moon is in its second quarter.

If you survive one coronary, the odds are three to one that you will not have another.

Some people eat oranges for vitamin C; some take tablets; others like fortified drinks. Not Captain Cook, though – he took three and a half tons of sauerkraut on one of his long-distance voyages.

You are literally one in a million if your IQ is over 180.

In 1932 an Italian boy was persuaded to sell one of his testicles to be implanted into a wealthy but less fortunate recipient.

A thousand schoolchildren given a course of vitamins were found to get just as many colds as a second thousand who received no medication at all.

After a severe illness in 1716, Lord Fermanagh started to take a posset of horse-dung every day as a tonic.

A 31-year-old man tried to commit suicide by holding a six-inch nail to his temple and banging it against a wall until it penetrated his skull. Then he pushed it in with his hands until only two inches was left showing. He made a complete recovery.

There are reckoned to be more than a million untreated syphilis cases in the United States.

In ancient Rome it was thought unlucky to pay a doctor's bill in full. The fates might think the patient over-satisfied and send him a fresh attack of his illness to teach him a lesson.

To Dr John Kellogg we owe not only breakfast cereals, but also the invention of peanut butter. He was a prominent health-food enthusiast and wrote 'Nuts May Save The Race'.

A Swedish psychoanalyst wrote extensively on the importance of charging high fees. He argued that in this way the analyst presents himself as a forthright individual who dares to be honest about money and is thus worthy of emulation. The fat fee was also an excellent outlet for the neurotic feelings of the masochistic patient, and a large bill did away with any potentially damaging 'humiliating sense of gratitude'.

Daniel Defoe in 1722 wrote of an Essex farmer who was living with his twenty-fifth wife, his two dozen previous ones having all died in childbirth. The man's 35-year-old son was at the time up to his fourteenth wife.

Ferrets can catch human colds.

One Russian woman's output of 69 children included 16 sets of twins, 7 of triplets and 4 sets of quadruplets.

Before the days of bottle-feeding, serious measures were needed to restore a mother's failing milk supply. Powdered earthworms, dried goat's udder, cuttlefish soup, shrimp heads, boiled sea-slugs, powdered silkworms in urine, or blow-fly maggots were reckoned to do the trick.

Charles I, Charles Lamb and Charles Darwin were all stutterers. So were Moses, Aristotle, Aesop and Virgil.

A new cure for drug addiction was announced in France. Twenty addicts were sent on an ocean cruise: thirteen were completely cured.

The anti-depressant drug iproniazid was derived from hydrazine, a component of rocket fuel.

Nineteenth-century dentures were sometimes made of celluloid, a fact which on at least one recorded occasion resulted in the teeth of a London clubland smoker catching fire.

Borborygmus, meaning flatulence, derives from a Greek word meaning 'I rumble'.

In the early 1800's, nurses at St George's hospital were paid £16 a year plus a shilling a day for board, a weekly allowance of 6lb of bread and two free pints of beer a day. Most of the larger hospitals ran their own breweries on the premises.

A medical professor sprayed water around a lecture room and asked his students to raise their hands as soon as the odour of water reached them. Seventy-five per cent did so.

At least one man is known to have become addicted to sodium bicarbonate, apparently because he liked the sensation of belching. By the time he went to hospital he was using half a pound a day.

Schridde found that 88 per cent of people who died from electrocution had made contact with the power-source through their left hands. As a safety measure, therefore, he advised those working near electrical equipment to keep their left hands in their pockets.

Nero ate vast quantities of leeks to improve his singing voice.

Roman villas had a special chamber known as a vomitorium, to which gourmets would retire at intervals during a banquet. After 'casting' they could return to the table and start all over again.

The medical kit issued to America's *Skylab* astronauts contained pills for travel sickness.

Joseph Harrod, a retired lock-keeper of Newark, decided to commit suicide. In twenty-four hours he twice tried to electrocute himself, twice cut his throat, and drank one-and-a-quarter bottles of whisky. Four days later he died of a cold.

A Swedish medical journal has reported that one in every seven hospital patients is given the wrong medication.

It was originally believed that the flow of mucus down the nose during a cold was fluid running out of the brain.

More animals are kept in drug-testing laboratories than in zoos.

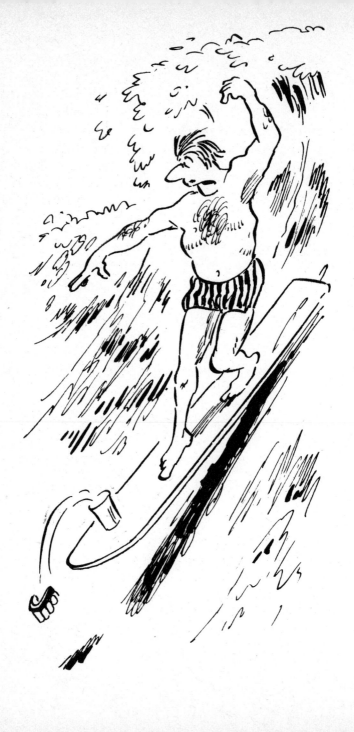

Surfing clubs in Brisbane recovered more than 200 sets of false teeth lost by surfers in Queensland's Gold Coast holiday area.

It was not until the Public Health Act of 1875 that any serious measures were taken to stop people pouring sewage into rivers. Thus, standing on a bridge over the River Cam early in her reign, Queen Victoria was moved to ask the Master of Trinity College: 'What are all those pieces of paper in the water?' The Master replied: 'Those, Your Majesty, are notices saying that bathing is forbidden.'

When the daughter of Emperor I Tsung of the Tang dynasty failed to recover from a fever, her father had the twenty most accomplished physicians in China beheaded.

Another American teenager becomes infected with VD every 11 minutes.

A woman of average size contains 9 gallons of water, enough carbon to make 9000 pencil leads, enough phosphorous for 8000 boxes of matches, enough iron for 5 nails, enough salt to fill 6 salt-cellars, and enough hydrogen to fill a balloon capable of lifting the body to the top of Snowdon.

Abortion and infanticide were so rife in ancient Greece and Rome that they had no need of contraceptives.

By the end of his course, a graduate in acupuncture will have stuck at least 10,500 needles into himself.

One out of five American men, and one out of four women, is ten per cent overweight.

Yoruba people cure childhood convulsions with *agbo tuto*. Young green tobacco leaves are the staple ingredient, activated by a 24-hour soak in urine. Gordon's gin may be added if the family can afford it.

In 1972 a nutritionist calculated that the population of Britain was about 100,000 tons overweight.

World Medicine reported that one of the most frustrating 'primary complications' of vasectomy was the wife's subsequent pregnancy.

Next time you feel ten years older than your age, spare a thought for the Brazilian child who died from the rare progeria disease. By the time he was six months old his adult teeth had not only appeared but were yellowing. At two years he had white hair going thin on top; and at ten he had the dry wrinkled skin and hardened arteries of an old man.

Each drop of blood travels nearly a mile a day round the human circulatory system.

Dr Anthony Iezzi, of St John's College, Cleveland, a leading American lecturer on medical ethics, warned an audience in Limerick that uncontrolled sex could only do harm to the quality of human life. He was speaking to 100 nuns.

Police began an investigation into the Family Church of Jesus in Great Yarmouth after two of the congregation drowned. The members of the sect believe they can walk on water.

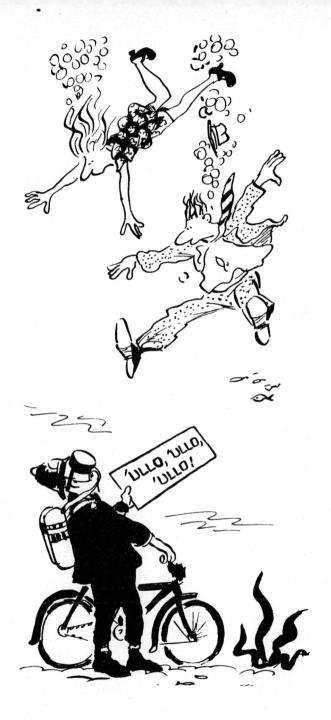

King Charles II was almost certainly killed by his own over-zealous physicians. During his final hours they administered sneezing powder; medicine prepared from extracts of human skull, peony and dissolved pearl; and an enema of beetroot, violets, antimony, linseed and cochineal. For the *coup de grâce* they bound the royal feet with a mix of Burgundy pitch and pigeon dung.

Radio-active bath-salts have been sold in the USA as an aid to rejuvenation.

There is no such thing as a 'Jewish nose'. A survey among Jewish New Yorkers revealed 57 per cent had flat noses, 14 per cent concave and 6.4 per cent flared. Only 22.3 per cent were 'typically' convex.

Six out of every ten babies are born before breakfast.

Diligent research quickly produced an effective contraceptive pill for men, but it turned users' eyeballs pink if they drank alcohol. Research continued.

Seventh-century medical etiquette dictated that doctors never wore purple or cut their hair too often.

Women are more likely than men to have arthritis, but less likely to have gout.

An American study of fatal heart attacks in Japan revealed that 80 per cent of the victims died immediately after, or during, extra-marital intercourse. And a third of them were drunk.

You are likely to spend 700 days, or one-fifth of your life, suffering from colds and other respiratory infections.

One of the reasons fewer Americans than you might expect die of lung cancer may be the extreme length of their dog-ends. The average American butt is 30.9 mm long, whereas the British smoker puffs on to within 18.7 mm of the tip. On the other hand the air in New York City is so polluted that even non-smokers suck in the equivalent of 40 cigarettes a day.

Following her own successful inoculation against smallpox, Catherine the Great ordered all Russian children to have the same treatment, and decreed that the first youngster to get a jab should be named Vaccinov. The first British child to be used as a guinea pig in this way had to be content with a free cottage.

There are 365 acupuncture points on the body, of which 21 are used for treating madness, 7 for impotence, 3 for sterility, and 1 each for nymphomania, drunkenness and boils.

Your mouth contains more bacteria than any other bodily orifice.

After analysing more than 250,000 weather reports, Dr Clarence Mills has established that human fertility reaches a peak at a temperature of 65 degrees f. During a heatwave in Kansas City, both fertility and desire dropped by 30 per cent.

One of the earliest recorded blood transfusions was attempted in the sixteenth century when a young Jewish doctor tried to restore the flagging vitality of Pope Innocent VIII with the blood of three boys. All participants but the doctor died shortly afterwards.

English soldiers at the Battle of Crécy in 1346 were so riddled with dysentery that the French called them the breechless, or bare-bottomed, army.

When it comes to birth control, no one can cap the Dutch. They opened the world's first clinic in 1882.

According to *Migraine News* there is a clear link between headaches and too much sex.

There is a good medical reason why corns are weather-prophets. When atmospheric pressure drops, the bursa (the sac containing the fluid that lubricates the joint) which is often inflamed by the corn and over-filled with fluid, can expand and apply angry pressure to the sore part of the toe.

Bananas are good for stopping diarrhoea, particularly in children.

Cold-cures submitted by members of the public to the Common Cold Research Unit at Salisbury have included: sniffing the mucus back instead of blowing the nose; avoiding dust from dance floors; standing naked in the draught from an electric fan; eating onion porridge; rubbing meths into bald heads; exposing yourself to teargas; growing a moustache; standing on your head under water, and having your house flattened by a V1 flying bomb.

King James the Sixth of Scotland and First of England became addicted to strong drink through the hooch he imbibed at the breast of an alcoholic wet nurse.

28

Canned music is piped into some American operating theatres to relax the surgeons.

A mere 1/200,000th oz of LSD is all that is needed to produce a reaction in the brain.

Americans spend $250,000,000 a year on phoney cures for arthritis.

The small print on the National Health Service form used in 1963 to set out general instructions to applicants for supplementary eye services was unreadable by anyone needing spectacles.

Two Chinese patients in a South African hospital were bleached so that they could transfer to a white ward.

It was the custom in the Celebes to fix fish-hooks on a sick man's feet, nose and navel to prevent his soul escaping.

A woman's efforts as a child-bearer are worth $10,000. This was the amount offered by a 45-year-old actuary, Leonard E. Goodfarb, in a Philadelphia newspaper advertisement for a woman prepared to have a baby for a childless couple. Mr Goodfarb was collecting information to help him put an actuarial valuation on a wife's services. He received so many replies from women eager to bear a child sired by someone else's husband that he had to go into hiding.

According to the ancient Greeks, there are two compartments in a womb – left for a girl and right for a boy.

A Los Angeles plastic surgeon found that men earned an average of $10,000 more in the year after cosmetic surgery than in the year before.

A large leech can absorb an ounce of blood at one sitting.

Roux, the German anatomist, had such a neurosis about the small size of his head that he ordered his brain to be removed and destroyed on his death. He was worried that it would be kept as an anatomical curiosity.

Inadequate sleep can slow a child's growth-rate by up to two-thirds.

A sleeping doctor had ready-made dreams supplied to him in a telepathy experiment. When the 'transmitter' formed a picture of a soldier blowing a bugle, the doctor dreamed of the Roman Army. Afterwards, as a treat, he was provided with a picture of Elizabeth Taylor.

If all the skins of all the people in Britain were laid out in the sun to dry, they would cover an area of 35 square miles. If the population of the world were skinned, the area covered would be 2260 square miles.

Police laboured in vain to discover the identity of a man brought into a Northern Ireland hospital. Interpreters spoke to him in ten different languages, but he made no response until someone tried him with Danish. It turned out he was an Irishman who had been to Denmark on holiday.

30

Australian Aboriginal babies are introduced to cosmetic surgery unusually early in life. Mother and father forcibly flatten young noses either by laying them face down on a hard surface, or by direct pressure with the palm of the hand.

Uninterrupted by exposure to radiation, a gene will pass unaltered through 50,000 human generations.

If you sleep three hours longer than usual, your reactions will be impaired in exactly the same way as if you had been deprived of rest.

Medicine in ancient Rome was regarded as a business fit only for slaves, freedmen and foreigners. Patricians were not allowed to practice it.

With 2500 fatalities a year, the sixth commonest cause of death in the United States is choking on food.

Medically speaking, a moron has an IQ of between 50 and 69, an imbecile has between 25 and 49, and an idiot between 0 and 24.

Frightened that the barbarians were breeding like rabbits while the Roman birthrate went down, Julius Caesar decreed that any Roman woman who died giving birth should be operated on to save the unborn child – hence 'Caesarian' operations.

Only four per cent of babies are born on the date predicted by the medical profession.

In 1967 Malaysian women were warned against trusting birth control pills made in Communist China. It was said their efficacy had yet to be proved.

Rado Pads, sold in America for between $7.50 and $30 each, were claimed to cure rheumatism, sinusitis and muscular ailments. They consisted of feather-ticking bags packed with plain crushed rock.

A man has survived 360 days on a diet of tap water.

Shipworkers loading tea-chests at Trincomalee, Sri Lanka, came across a consignment of jam, and loading stopped while the men consumed an average of two jars each. The shift then resumed, but broke up in disorder when the vessel's lavatory proved disastrously inadequate for the workers' sudden dramatic needs. The 'jam' was a laxative.

You can inhale as much benzpyrene while barbecuing a steak as you can from smoking 700 untipped cigarettes.

South African Mrs Janni Swanepoel has just 'retired' after giving birth to her twenty-ninth child, a feat inspired by remarks made in 1965 by Mr Botha, the Minister for Bantu Development. 'The Minister told us to populate the country because the blacks were outnumbering us', she said. 'I decided this is just what we shall do – I've never been sorry.' Alas Mr Botha – no father figure he – now explains that his words were misreported all those years ago, and silly Mrs Swanepoel's labours have all been due to a misunderstanding.

Women need more sleep than men.

A famous tonic contains such minute quantities of vitamins and minerals that a cup of cocoa has four times more iron than the recommended dose of the tonic; half-a-pint of London tapwater has fifty times more calcium; and one chip has an identical quantity of Vitamin C.

A prescription sold at the time of the Great Plague specified 'the brains of a young man that hath died a violent death, together with its membranes, arteries, veins, nerves and all the pith of the backbone, bruising these in a stone mortar 'til they become a kind of pap, then putting in as much of spirits of wine as will cover the breadth of three fingers, and digesting for half a year in horse dung'. To be taken once a day, with water.

Dr Erwin O. Strassman of Houston, Texas, studied 717 childless women and found that, broadly speaking, the bigger the breasts the smaller the IQ.

A British Army officer's big toe is worth £30 more than a corporal's, according to the Schedule of Specific Minor Injuries published in the *London Gazette*. Index-fingers are good rank-pullers as well. The corporal's meagre digit is valued at £65 less than his superior's more elegant organ.

British male alcoholics outnumber females by four to one.

Half of Britain's population has lost all its natural teeth by middle age.

A typist working in a busy office wastes 20 per cent of her energy fighting against the noise. An executive wastes 30 per cent.

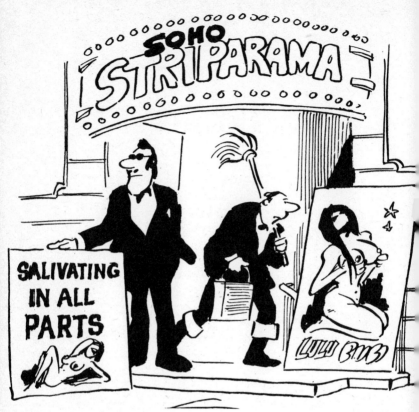

The inhabitants of Greater London produce about three million gallons of saliva every twenty-four hours.

Nicholas Wood, the 'Great Eater of Kent', once ate a whole sheep at a sitting. His chronicler, Taylor, adds: 'I thinke he left the skin, the wool, the hornes, and the bones'. At Lord Wooton's table the Eater had 84 rabbits at one go, and on another occasion 30 dozen pigeons. His usual breakfast was 18 yards of black pudding.

34

Constant emphasis on sexual performance has been found to cause loss of virility in Swedish men.

VD is second only to measles as a health hazard in Barnet.

As a deterrent against hairy faces, bearded lawyers in the sixteenth century were charged extra for taking dinner in their Inns of Court.

A research group at Michigan University medical school made a set of dentures containing six radio transmitters to broadcast all the sounds made in the wearer's mouth while he ate, drank, smoked and slept.

Fresh gladiator blood was drunk in Rome as a cure for epilepsy.

If one identical twin is homosexual, his brother nearly always is too. If he's a non-identical twin, there is a 50 per cent chance that his brother will be 'normal'.

Fashionable psychology has firmly cast the cigarette in the role of nipple substitute. Support for this theory has been provided by research showing a direct link between the ability to stop smoking and the age of weaning. Those who could not kick the habit were weaned at an average age of 4.7 months; those who gave up easily, however, had not been deprived of the real thing until they were 8 months old.

Minnesota Department of Health statistics showed that deaths from arteriosclerosis rose to a peak in January, suicides peaked in May, and accidental deaths in July and August.

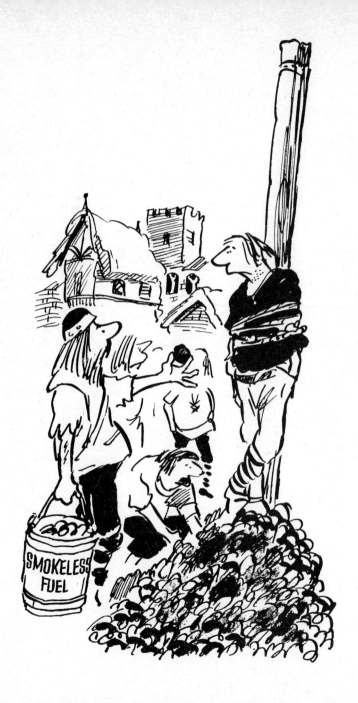

As long ago as 1273, coal fires were banned in London as a potential health hazard. It is recorded that at least one persistent offender was put to death for his disobedience.

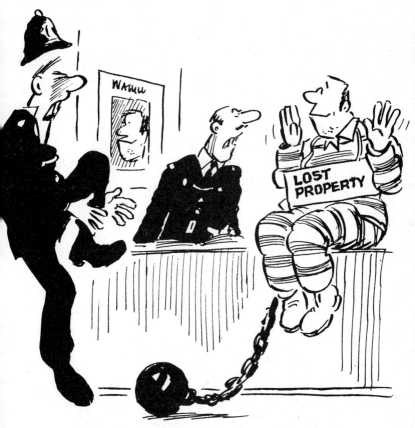

Police Constable Kenneth King suffered a broken toe when a ball and chain fell on his foot at Full Street police station, Derby. A police spokesman explained after the accident that the ball and chain was 'lost property'.

One in five of Birmingham's policemen is married to a nurse.

There used to be little need for dentists in the East Indies. It was customary to file the teeth down to the gums as part of the ceremonial at weddings and puberty, and during mourning.

The network of nerves in your brain contains more possible connections than there would be in a universal telephone exchange supplying a telephone to every individual in the world.

When seized with a compulsion to smoke, the members of an anti-smoking organisation in Los Angeles can dial a number and listen to a recording of a man having a coughing fit.

Non-worshipping Americans have been found to have twice as much chance of suffering heart attacks as churchgoers.

Following the advice of one of his doctors, Louis xv forced Madame de Pompadour to eat animal testicles to cure her frigidity.

Five-month-old babies can distinguish between angry and happy faces.

Some of the most intimate data recorded in Masters and Johnson's *Human Sexual Responses* was obtained with a transparent plastic penis containing a movie lens.

Men go through emotional cycles similar to menstruation.

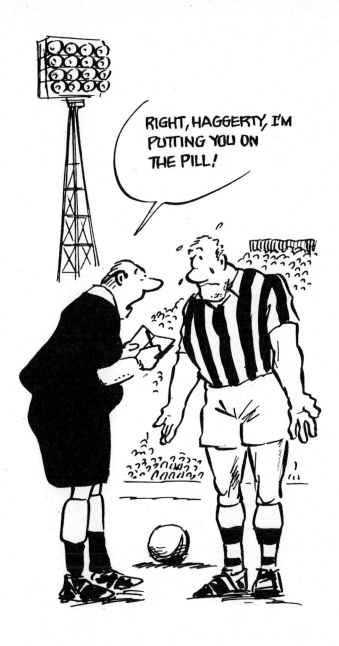

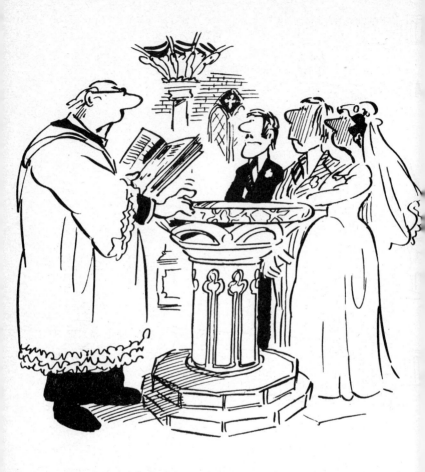

More British babies are born in the sixth month after marriage than at any other time.

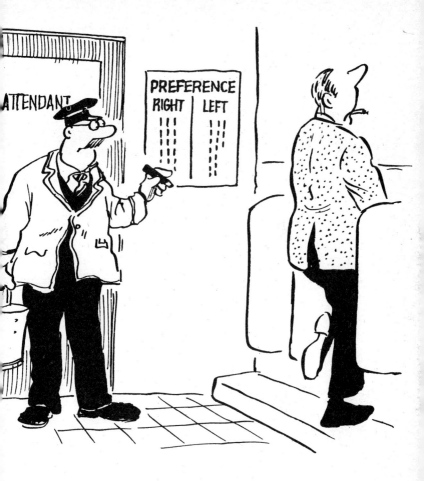

Most people stand on one leg. An English survey in 1953 showed that 1432 people out of 1710 stood with their weight on one leg at a time. They constantly fidgeted from left to right, but hardly ever rested on both together.

When Dr Albert Abrams died in 1923 he left a fortune of two million dollars from sales of his Dynamic Abramic Pole and reflexaphones which, he insisted, could diagnose any illness from a single drop of a patient's blood. A jealous rival once sent him some rooster's blood and was duly informed that the patient was suffering from malaria, diabetes, cancer and two separate venereal diseases.

The world's doctors are kept up to date by a deluge of more than 6000 specialist medical journals. Only a small minority, however, have the panache of an American publication called *Medical Confessions*, whose headlines in one issue included: You'll Never Be a Doctor's Wife; The Teenage Boy With a Girl's Body; I'll Give You a New Face; His Lung is Full of Cancer; and Abnormal Sex Demands – What Are They?

An 85-year old Iranian and his 69-year-old wife became the parents of twins in 1967.

Midwives were unknown to the Incas. Mothers took just enough time off to deliver their own babies and wash them in a stream before immediately resuming normal household duties.

Sylvester Graham, a modern pioneer of vegetarianism, believed spice-eating caused madness, tea brought delirium tremens and meat 'inflamed the baser propensities'. He lived only to 57, however, having a sceptical wife who made a point of cooking tempting dishes to lead him off the straight and narrow.

42

When a general retired as head of the US Chemical Corps he visited each installation to say goodbye to his men. At one base an elaborate demonstration was staged in which several thousand guinea pigs were satisfactorily exterminated with nerve gas. Impressed, the general remarked : 'Now we know what to do if we ever go to war against guinea pigs'.

It was an ancient Chinese belief that sperm was stored in the brain. As each man was reckoned to have only a limited supply, ejaculation was permitted only when a son was wanted.

The table manners of a boy named Tom suffered permanent and spectacular impairment in 1895 when he seared his mouth with scalding clam chowder. It burned his gullet so badly that it became blocked. All attempts to unblock it failed, so a surgeon set out to fix a by-pass tube around the obstruction. But, before the operation was complete, the patient's condition deteriorated so rapidly that the doctor had to make do with a rush job – an inch-and-a-half hole in the boy's stomach. When Tom recovered he learned to feed himself by chewing his food and spitting it through a funnel and rubber tube into the hole. He ate twice a day and had to wait five hours between meals for his stomach to empty.

About one calorie of energy is needed to read a page of 650 words, roughly the same as the energy from a tomato or a cup of black coffee.

In 1975 it was reported that 200,000 British children under the age of eleven were on tranquillisers.

Drink is no longer the curse of the working classes. Those most likely to succumb to alcoholism are officers in the armed forces, journalists, actors, commercial travellers and publicans.

The first recorded use of chloroform as an anaesthetic was in 1847 when one of the recipients exclaimed 'I'm an angel' as sleep bore her off.

Before the supply dried up, inhaling the breath of young virgins was thought to have wide-ranging curative effects.

The nasal passages are lined with erectile tissue similar to the penis. Ham's *Histology*, a textbook widely used in American medical schools, quotes the case of a sixteenth-century youth who sneezed every time he saw a pretty girl. None of which might have surprised the ancient Indian lawmakers of Manu, who decreed that adulterers should be punished by having their noses cut off.

The British blood transfusion services dispense more than 163,250 entire bodiesful of blood every year.

Crushed brick soaked in olive oil was administered in the eighteenth century as a cure for gout.

Joseph Lister pioneered antiseptic dressings by pouring impure, undiluted carbolic acid straight into the wound of 11-year-old James Greenless, who had a compound fracture of the left leg. How Master Greenless expressed his gratitude at the time is not recorded.

There is new hope for those worried about their cholesterol intake. Kangaroo meat is cholesterol-free.

When Henry II of France had his eye pierced by a splinter from a jousting lance, his surgeons tried to find the best way of treating him by having four criminals beheaded and thrusting broken truncheons into their eyes.

If all the bits of tube cut out in Indian vasectomy operations were shipped to England and laid end to end, they would stretch from London to Birmingham.

The religious relics at the shrines of St Ursula at Cologne and St Rosalia at Palermo retained their alleged healing powers even after the skeletal remains of 11,000 virgins at the former were found to be those of men, and the bones of St Rosalia were discovered to belong to a goat.

According to Samuel Sharp, a surgeon at Guy's Hospital in the 1700s: 'In the hospitals of London, bugs are frequently a greater evil to the patient than the malady for which he seeks an hospital'. Things have changed nowadays, of course, though not as much as you might expect. One in seven patients still picks up a new infection during his stay in hospital.

The human nose is the only instrument capable of measuring smell – a fact acknowledeged by ICI at Billingham, who cut public complaints of bad smells by 75 per cent by appointing a specially-trained nose-patrol. The sniffers' duties included making regular reconnaissance sorties as well as investigating complaints of every odour.

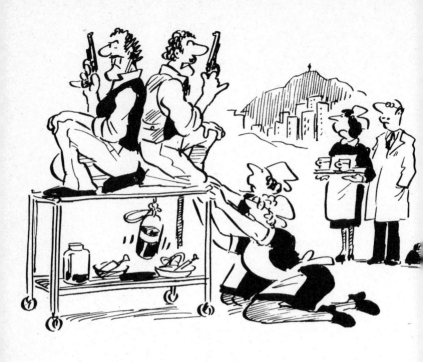

Duelling is legal in Uruguay provided both parties are registered blood donors.

Men nearly always have erections while they dream, even the elderly and those who have had intercourse immediately before dropping off. The degree of tumescence is reduced during anxious dreams.

A three-year-old girl admitted to hospital in 1974 was found to have eaten ice lollipops made from Valium syrup.

Matthew Buchinger, born in Germany in 1674, had no hands, feet, legs or thighs, and was twenty-nine inches tall. His arms were 'more resembling of fins of fish than arms of men'. Nevertheless, he was advertised as able to make a pen and write as quick and well as any writing master, to draw faces to the life, and coats of arms, pictures and flowers, to thread a fine needle very quickly, and to shuffle a pack of cards and deal them 'very swift'. He could play a dulcimer as well as any musician, and did 'many surprising things with cups and balls, giving the curious great satisfaction thereby'. He could play skittles, shave himself, and 'dance a hornpipe in a Highland dress as well as any man without legs ... and many other things too tedious to insert'.

People fall asleep more readily when the atmospheric pressure is low.

One way of overcoming a transplant patient's tendency to 'reject' new tissue is to choose a new organ so genetically alien as to completely baffle his body's defence system. Hence pigs' kidneys have successfully been put into humans.

Cow pats, being soft and heat-engendering, make effective poultices and have been applied with success for tumours, ulcers, breast cancer, boils, pneumonia and whitlows.

In 1970 a young Californian drug addict was charged with eating his friendly welfare worker.

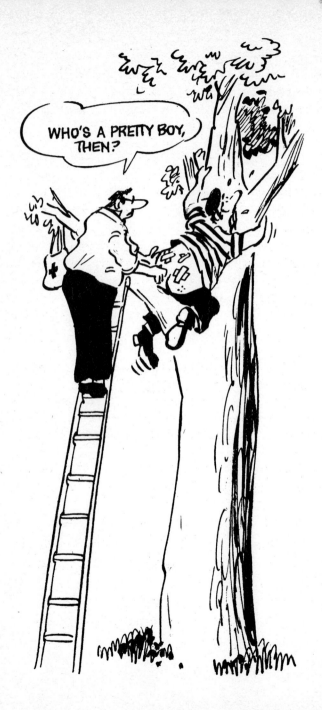

A doctor in Tarrasa, Spain, was called to a tree to give emergency aid to a weekend hunter who had climbed into the branches to try and lure birds within range. His twittering noises at least convinced another hunter, who shot him.

The trouble with liquid silicone injections, as one plastic surgeon lamented, is that 'a lot of the stuff disappears. You don't know where it's going to go, but it always travels'. So one middle-aged would-be beauty found to her cost. She had her frown-line filled out with liquid silicone and the effect pleased her for a while. One morning, however, she woke up to find her nose stretching all the way across her eyelids and wider by an inch around the nostrils.

A contest was staged at the Royal Court of Salermo in the early middle ages to see which of two physicians had the greater knowledge of drugs. The first man successfully to poison the other was declared the winner and was later appointed Bishop of Amiens.

Blood from fresh corpses is used in Russia for transfusions.

Following Maggie Dickson's hanging at Musselburgh, a band of medical students tried to cut the body down and take it away for dissection. Friends of the deceased resisted and there ensued a pitched battle which ceased only when Mrs Dickson unexpectedly stirred and came to life. She lived another 30 years, known always as 'half-hangst' Maggie Dickson.

Five medical students were sent down from the Hebrew University at Jerusalem after one of them accepted a dare to eat a slice of human brain. When the news leaked out, four people who had been intending to leave their bodies to the university revoked their wills, and a heart patient fled the Hadassah Hospital in terror of what might lie in store for him if he died.

In a public health prosecution in 1347, two men were charged with piping their excrement into a neighbour's cellar. The offence was not noticed until the cellar overflowed.

Peru holds at least one version of the world junior childbirth record. In 1939 a girl in that country had her first menstrual period at eight months and was delivered of a live baby, by Caesarian section, at the age of five. The younger child weighed 5lb 13oz. The *Rangoon People's Daily*, however, has entered a challenge with the reported pregnancy of a three-year-old Burmese girl.

Five hundred million humans carry hookworm.

Doctors had a quieter time than usual on the opening day of the Italian shooting season in 1974. Only six hunters died – four shot by other marksmen and two dying from heart attacks after successfully potting hares. Forty others were wounded.

According to official statistics, the most dangerous room in the French home is the bedroom, 'where 44.5 per cent of all accidents occur'.

50

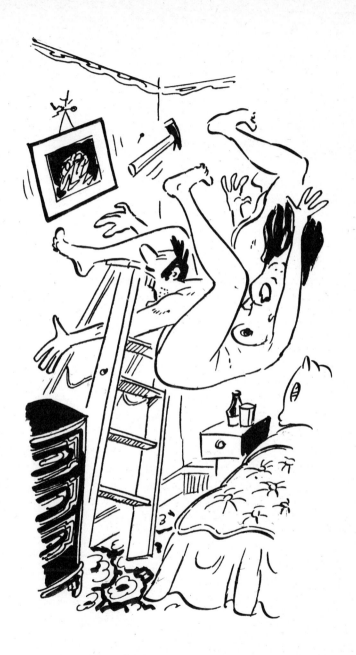

The mummified body of an Egyptian who died 3000 years ago was admitted to a Durham hospital with six slipped discs, stones in the kidney and the earliest known example of a prosthetic hand.

Cigarettes kill more people than all accidents, infectious diseases, suicides, alcohol and cancer of the stomach put together.

The respected *New Orleans Medical and Surgical Journal* described in 1851 the newly discovered disease of drapetomania – a form of insanity found only in Negro slaves and characterised by their desire to run away from their masters.

Lady Coventry was the first victim to cosmetics. She died on October 1, 1760, from the effects of regularly painting her face with white lead.

Doctors at a hospital in Framington, Massachusetts, had a ward converted into a bar after it was discovered that regular beer made patients more responsive to treatment. The project was so successful that they applied for a research grant to cover some of the costs.

An article in an 1878 issue of the *British Medical Journal* maintained that the proximity of a menstruating woman had caused a ham to spoil.

A doctor listing commonly-occurring dream objects which psychoanalysts take to be symbolic of sexual organs or activities found 102 symbols for penis and 55 for coitus.

A thief broke into Manchester Royal Infirmary and stole 800 assorted glass eyes.

52

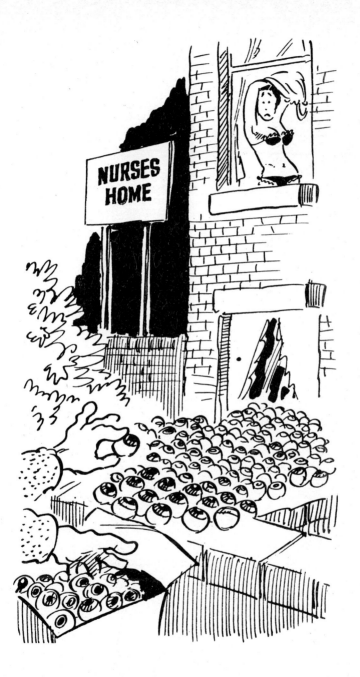

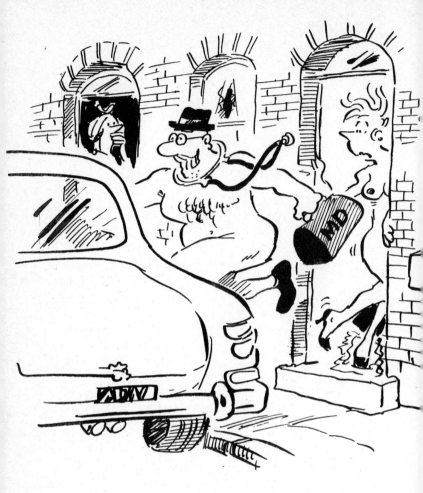

A Hampshire Medical Officer of Health reported that
'General Practitioners were responsible for 80 per cent
of the hospital confinements of mothers'.

It was not easy for Chinese in the early centuries AD to find the best doctor in town, for his premises would inevitably be dimly lit and obscure. An Imperial order obliged every physician to shine a lantern outside his house for every one of his patients who had died from other than natural causes.

The earliest stethoscopes were carried inside doctors' top hats.

Eighteenth-century surgeon John Hunter is best remembered for his observation of the effects of castration on cockerels' combs, and for his experimental research into the nature of venereal disease. In 1767 he injected himself with pus from a patient with gonorrhoea, and not only proved that this disease can be transmitted but also accidentally infected himself with syphilis, from which he is believed to have died.

The first X-ray picture is said to have been of Roentgen's wife's hand. She accidentally leaned on a photographic plate while inquiring her husband's reasons for his lateness at supper.

In America each year more than twice as many psychiatrists commit suicide as mental hospital patients.

Aristotle believed food was 'cooked' in the heart and transformed into blood.

The Church opposed use of the first effective treatment for syphilis on the grounds that the disease was a just punishment for immorality.

Chinese and Japanese babies are born with blue bruises on their bottoms.

A hiccups epidemic forced a school in Vienna to close for several weeks.

More female suicides, accidents and crimes occur during the first few days of the menstrual cycle.

If you think the Sphinx looks as if she has a bad odour under her nose, you're probably right. The Egyptians considered garlic so energy-rich that they maintained the slaves building the pyramids on a diet that consisted of little but garlic and onions. At least it made them *smell* strong.

Between 1.30 am and 5.30 am last night you moved in your sleep about 40 times. Unless you are an insomniac, of course, in which case you will have shifted position at least 70 times.

To find the best spot in Baghdad to build a new hospital, Rhazes, a tenth-century Persian physician, suspended bits of raw meat on a variety of sites. He chose the place where the flesh took longest to putrefy, reasoning that this ground must have the healthiest air.

The world's medical research journals are published at the rate of three a minute.

Though barbers took care of surgery, it was the English blacksmith who added to his income by bone-setting.

A nine-stone woman exerts a pressure of 1200 lb per square inch on her thigh bones in the mere act of walking. The thighs of pole-vaulters have to be able to withstand 20,000 lb per square inch on landing.

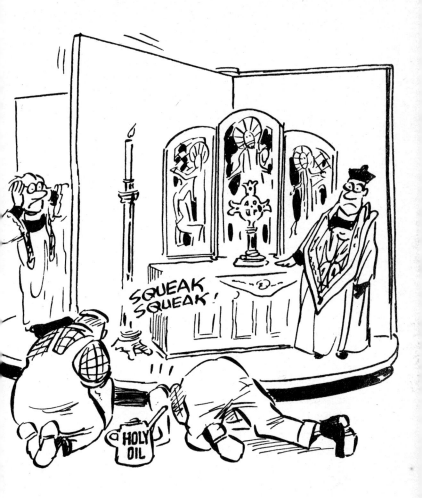

SQUEAK
SQUEAK!

HOLY
OIL

The chapel of a new hospital in Cumberland was
equipped with three separate altars on a revolving
Palladium-style platform so that it could be used in
turn for Church of England, Roman Catholic and Free
Church services.

57

The earliest baby's feeding bottles were cows' horns fitted with heifers' teats.

You have got approximately 2,500,000 sweat glands.

If you pulled the plug out of an 11.5 stone man and drained all the water out of him, he would reduce immediately to 4.75 stones.

A Nigerian witch doctor was sentenced to death for shooting dead a client while testing a bullet-proof charm.

Preventive medicine was a particular speciality of the celebrated Dutch doctor, Boerhaave. When he was called to an orphanage at Haarlem to attend to an outbreak of fits, he at once ordered fires to be lit all over the building and suspended branding irons in the flames. Then he assembled the children and promised to brand the first one to show signs of convulsion. Not a twitch occurred.

Two men taken to the medical centre at Heathrow Airport close to death had each swallowed 24 rubber contraceptives containing liquid cannabis. They may or may not have had something to do with the strange condition of an 18-year-old Swedish girl in Eilat, Israel, who gave birth to a wombful of opium – two nylon bags containing some 100 grams.

A recent redevelopment plan for part of Knightsbridge was turned down because of underground plague-pits, which could cause another outbreak if exposed. The plague virus takes 1000 years to die.

58

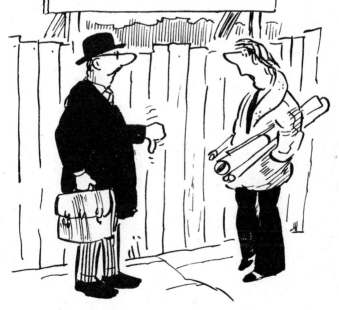

Musically untutored listeners recognise melodies best with the left ear, but the right side works best for connoisseurs. Right-handed people tend to pick up low notes in the left ear and high in the right, but left-handers show no defnite preferences.

Leopold Auenbrugger, of Vienna, was the first doctor to advocate in 1761 the now time-honoured practice of tapping a patient's chest and back to aid diagnosis. Quick off the mark, the medical world ignored his suggestion for a century.

Eating a lot of liquorice can lead to high blood pressure.

Most contraceptive pills are made from substances found in the Mexican yam and the urine of pregnant mares.

Police officers are the most persistent wife-batterers, said Mrs Erin Pizzey, founder of the Women's Aid organisation.

Phineas Gage, an American railroad worker in the 1840s, provided doctors with much useful information about the workings of the brain. When a crowbar was driven through his head during blasting operations, it produced only a mild personality-change.

Americans who have their bodies frozen and stored at −196°C until cures have been found for their diseases have been advised to take enough money into cold storage with them to pay their doctor's fees when they are eventually thawed out and restored to health.

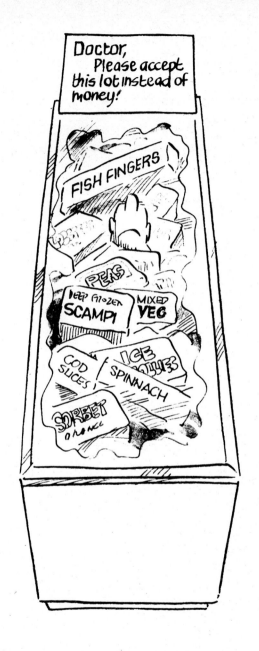

Blue blood is found in only two circumstances. Either you're being asphyxiated or you are a member of the lobster family.

A Nuremberg woman was taken to hospital with suspected brain damage after trying to smuggle a frozen chicken out of a supermarket under her hat. She fainted at the check-out.

A committee of experts appointed by the British Medical Association in the 1930s to assess the nutritional state of the nation set their 'standard' slightly below the minimum official dietary requirements of the Scottish prison service. After they had found that 20 per cent of the population lived at or below this level, the Ministry of Health rejected their report on the grounds that they had set too high a standard.

Animals injected with strong doses of nicotine become noticeably more intelligent, but soon die.

The suicide rate for men is about twice that for women.

Police in Pontoise, France, were worried about the condition of a man who had tried to kiss a girl in the street and then run away. She had bitten off his tongue.

More people are kicked to death by donkeys than die in flying accidents.

For more than 500 years the standard work on uroscopy – the study of urine – was Gilles de Corbeil's *Carmina de Urinarum*. It was written, after the fashion of the time, entirely in verse.

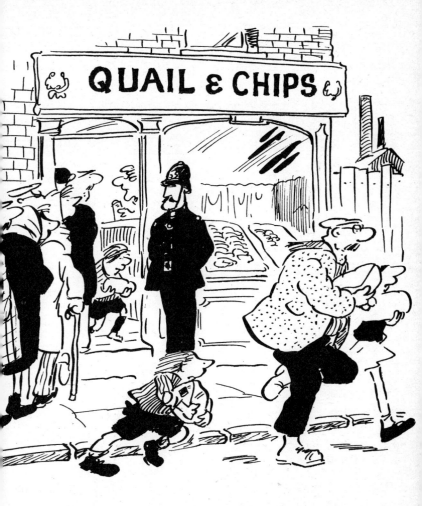

The coronation of Edward VII had to be postponed at two days' notice for the removal of the royal appendix. As a result, many poor families feasted on the 2500 quails and hundreds of chickens, sturgeons and partridge intended for the coronation banquet.

Planning blight is explained. Grandiose, though rational, schemes are often a symptom of the terminal stages of syphilis.

Your brain uses about as much power as a 10-watt electric bulb.

Two people were treated for monkey bites in Bognor Regis during the summer of 1972, one more than in 1971.

In 1870 the principal of the Harvard Medical School said written examinations could not be given to his students as most of them could not write well enough.

One of the Salem witches hanged on the testimony of Deliverance Hobbs was accused of bewitching a horse, a roast pig and a canoe.

Although the Assyrians practised ritual circumcision, they were humane enough to anaesthetise the boys beforehand. They choked them into insensibility.

According to Seymour Hersh's *Chemical and Biological Warfare*, the United States Chemical Corps was in the late 1960s looking into the possibility of spreading bubonic plague bacilli to Siberia on the feet of migrating geese.

A helping of raw Brussels sprouts containing 130 milligrams of vitamin C has only one-tenth that amount when cooked.

In Mauritius, 37 babies were born for every 1000 of the island's population in 1900. In 1966 the figure was exactly the same.

King George IV, as Prince Regent, often had himself bled so that he would look pale and elegant.

Three thousand of Britain's 97,000 postmen suffered from dog-bites in 1968.

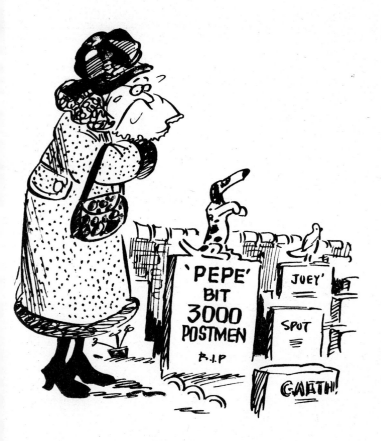

'PEPE'
BIT
3000
POSTMEN
R.I.P

'JUEY'

SPOT

GARTH

Dan Dale Alexander's *Arthritis and Common Sense* has sold more than half a million copies since it was first published in 1951. 'This book is the greatest since the Holy Bible in the opinion of people who write to me,' Alexander said, 'and I am willing to accept that opinion.' He claims the symptoms of arthritis include: dry skin, dandruff, ridged finger-nails, wrinkles, itchy nose or rectum, buzzing in the ears, varicose veins, sterility and an absence of ear-wax.

Fashionable Regency bucks liked to wear dentures made from 'Waterloo teeth', pulled from corpses on the battle field. Later, teeth from the American Civil War were shipped to England by the barrel.

Florence Nightingale thought the ideal nurse was a girl of 'the small farmers' class – physically strong, endowed with common sense, energetic and cheerful'. She reckoned a nurse could pick up all she needed to know in six months.

Elegant gentry of the eighteenth century used to wear 'plumpers', cork pads in the cheeks to fill out the hollows left by rotten teeth.

A popular medicine in the 1830s was Dr Mile's Extract of Tomato. The recipe survives, only today it is known as tomato ketchup.

The Institute of Baths Management reported that 55 of the men recruited as attendants at public swimming pools in 1974 were morally unsuitable, 9 sexually assaulted customers, 27 hit people, got drunk or took drugs on duty, 55 left their pools unattended and 150 couldn't swim.

66

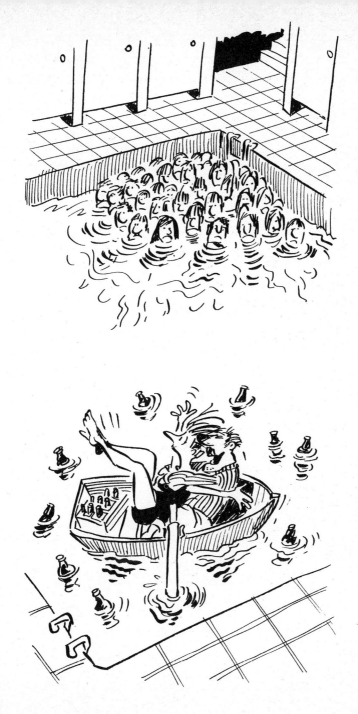

The 1937 edition of the *United States Dispensary* listed 3090 drugs. Within 30 years, 2470 of these had been proved useless.

Your normal daily output of urine is around 1.5 litres.

Before anaesthesia, surgeons were more concerned with the duration than with the intensity of pain during an operation. The best of them boasted they could have a leg off in under a minute, and a certain Robert Liston once managed it in 28 seconds.

The Fiji gold miners' trade union complained that members were too weary at the end of the day to oblige their wives, and demanded a 30-minute sex break. Bachelors were to be excluded, however: 'We don't want to overdo it.'

Tobacco was thought to have wide powers of healing in the sixteenth century. Its leaves were applied to wounds and smoke blown up the rectum.

American plastic surgeons were recently charging $1000 for a thigh-lift operation, in which the skin on both legs is pulled up, tucked in and sewn into a crease round the groin. Somewhat cheaper was the insertion of cosmetic testicles. These cost $19 the pair, installation extra.

Most people sweat about 30 oz of fluid a day.

The average size of Glaswegian children decreased in 1970.

Miss Sigrid Hemse, of Gotland, Sweden, announced her intention to sue the psycho-kineticist Uri Geller for her unwanted pregnancy. She said Mr Geller's unusual powers caused her contraceptive device to bend when she and her fiancé, Mr Sven Malmo, made love while watching him on television.

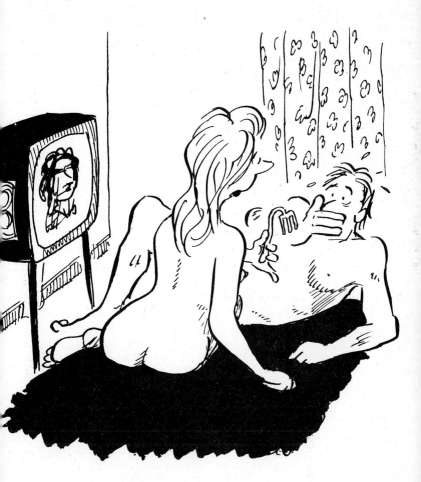

Europe's first skin bank opened at the Industrial Accidents Clinic at Ludwigshafen/Oggersheim, West Germany, in March 1973. Pieces of skin 5 cm x 20 cm are peeled from donors and preserved in liquid nitrogen.

In 1702 John Marten wrote enthusiastically about an impregnated linen condom which would prevent venereal infection. He declined to reveal the formula, however, 'lest it give encouragement to the lewd'.

Roughly 20 per cent of British cosmetic operations to remove bags from under the eyes, and 15 per cent of face-lifts, are done on men.

A report filed with the United Nations in 1952 accused America of attacking Korea and China with cholera-infected clams and anthrax-infected feathers; lice, fleas, mosquitoes, rabbits and other small animals dosed with plague and yellow fever; and other, more run-of-the-mill, items such as germ-loaded lavatory paper, envelopes and fountain pens.

Foul stinks were held to be an efficacious protection against the plague. Thus many a prudent Englishman was moved to share his bed with a goat and to spend as many of his wakeful hours as he could with his head thrust deep in the privy, greedily sucking in its life-preserving fumes.

It was the opinion of Erasmus that any nobleman who failed to contract syphilis was 'ignobilis et rusticans', or a base oaf.

British soldiers in the Second World War had their underwear impregnated with DDT to give immunity from lice. The enemy were not similarly protected, which possibly contributed to their demise.

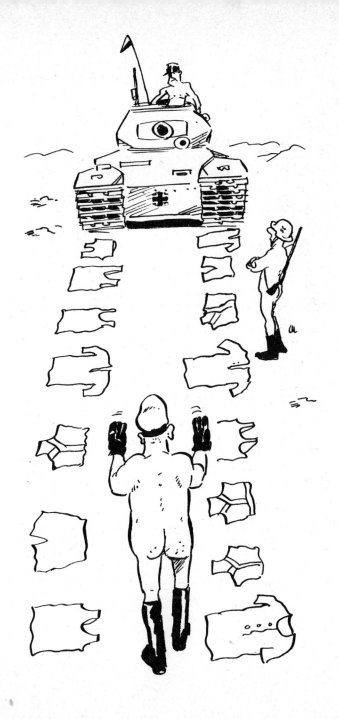

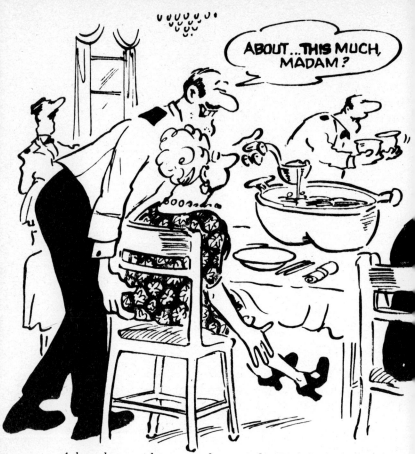

A lunch served to members of the Welsh Arts Council Sculpture Committee was served up on crockery moulded by sculptress Beryl Cheame from bits of her own body. 'I got the idea during a dinner party', she explained. 'All at once I realised what a marvellous food container the body is.' She used her breasts to mould the soup dishes, and her stomach for the plates. 'Later I added a casserole which was formed around a cast of my behind.'

72

A modern 80-year-old European has a shorter life-expectancy than his counterpart of 1805.

The maximum speed of air passing through the nostrils during normal breathing is about Force Two on the Beaufort Scale – ten feet per second, described as a light breeze.

A doctors' surgery in Sandwich, Kent, has 'The Butchery' as its address.

The word 'testis' derives from the Latin for 'witness'. Men were not allowed to testify in court unless both were present.

A recent American diet fad consisted almost exclusively of whole-grain cereal and tea. Its promoters claimed it would cure more than 80 ailments ranging from dandruff to cancer. In practice it was ideal for obesity but little help for the scurvy from which its stricter adherents invariably suffered.

The first war in which wounds took a greater toll than disease was probably the Russo-Japanese war of 1904-5.

Sussex suffered an outbreak of bubonic plague in 1910.

There were many cases of unhealthy seepage from medieval privies into wells. But this wasn't the only peril inherent in cesspools, as the unlucky Richard the Baker found out. He disappeared through the rotten planks of his latrine and 'drowned monstrously in his own excrement'.

The Chenchu of India believe that nocturnal intercourse means blind children.

Before the invention of obstetric forceps, the instruments commonly used to aid childbirth were spoons, knives and farm tools, of which the most popular was the thatcher's hook.

In 1972 a medical student in Marseilles decided one of his tutors was not up to scratch, so he shot him. 'He was a hindrance to my medical career', he explained afterwards.

Monks were forbidden to practise medicine in 1212 because too many of them were forsaking their religious obligations in the monasteries for the life of luxury provided by their rich patients.

You constantly shed particles of skin, amounting to one entire outer layer every 28 days.

Bunarr Macfadden was a dynamic proponent of vegetarianism who ran a travelling health show in which he and his wife stripped to their scanties and performed mighty muscular feats. For the finale, Mrs Macfadden leaped rump-first on to her husband's belly. It was Macfadden's stated belief that, during depressions, poor people should be deep-frozen and put into storage to be thawed out when business picked up again.

Quinine used to be called Jesuit Powder.

A man's neck has seven vertebrae. So does a giraffe's.

A 56-year-old Pole died in Stoke-on-Trent from choking on a garlic clove he left in his mouth overnight to ward off dracula-like monsters.

74

Your general muscular strength is at its peak around the age of 25, and diminishes slowly afterwards. Different muscles decline at different rates. Those of the back and hand take only until the age of 37 to revert to what they were at 20. Wrist and elbow don't reach this point of decay until 45; fingers take until 50. The general muscular strength of a 65-year-old man is roughly equal to that of a 25-year-old woman.

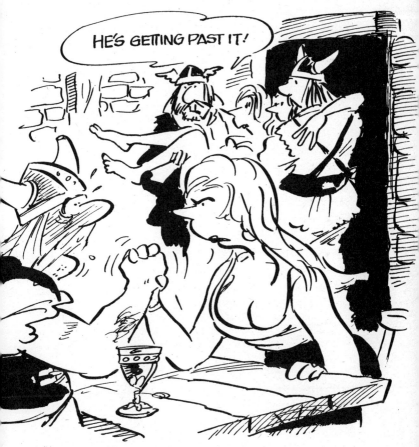

In 1882, George Littlewood walked 531 miles in six days.

Allied Intelligence in the Second World War feared that German V-1 flying bombs would carry warheads containing botulinus toxin, half a pound of which, properly distributed, would kill everyone in the world. Canada sent 235,000 doses of antidote to London, and self-inoculating syringes were issued to 117,500 Allied troops in readiness for the cataclysm. There was considerable relief when the first V-1 to arrive contained merely high explosive.

Ten thousand artificially-inseminated women give birth in America every year.

Cough medicine dispensed by St Bartholemew's Hospital, London, in the nineteenth century, benefited children's pockets rather than their health. The syrup was so sweet the children were able to do a brisk trade selling it for a penny per bottle to an old lady in Smithfield. She used it to make jam tarts.

There are about three million bacteria in every ounce of human faeces.

Peter the Great, first Tsar of Russia, proclaimed a tax on beards and eventually decreed that any such growth appearing within his kingdom should be shaved with a blunt razor or plucked out, one hair at a time, with pincers.

It was thought indecent for Chinese women to undress in front of doctors, who therefore had to provide ivory statuettes on which the ladies could point out where they felt unwell.

76

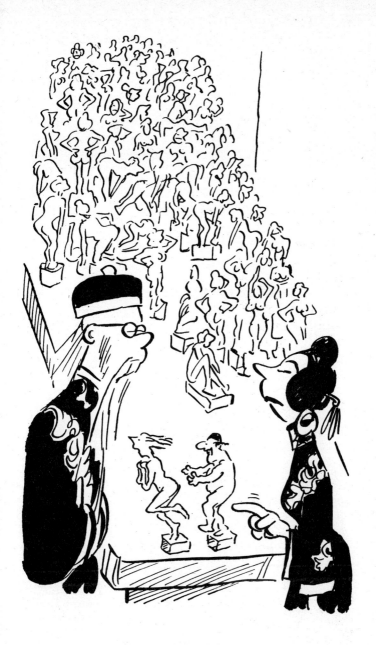

A 55-year-old woman was awarded £10,000 damages for the loss of her sex-life as a result of a bingo accident. She fell off her chair. Her husband received £50 for loss of consortium.

Human blood cost £125 a gallon in the United States during 1974; Chanel No. 5 perfume was £650.

The front page of the *Daily Mirror* requires a reading age of 12. Its editorial requires a reading age of 13, the same as the front page of the *Daily Telegraph*. The reading age required to understand the terms of the average hire purchase agreement is too high to be calculated.

Bacon's Cordial Essence of Russian Rhubarb was a famous purgative.

Sixteenth-century Britons were forbidden to beat their wives after 10 pm.

Chinese doctors inoculated against smallpox by collecting scabs from the drying pustules of someone with a mild case of the disease, grinding them to a powder and blowing it up the new patient's nostrils.

Platearius wrote in the twelfth century that tooth decay was caused by worms. 'When the teeth are washed with warm water and the water is poured into a vessel, the worms can be seen swimming about.'

In athletic events beyond 400 metres, the longer the race the shorter on average is the runner who wins it.

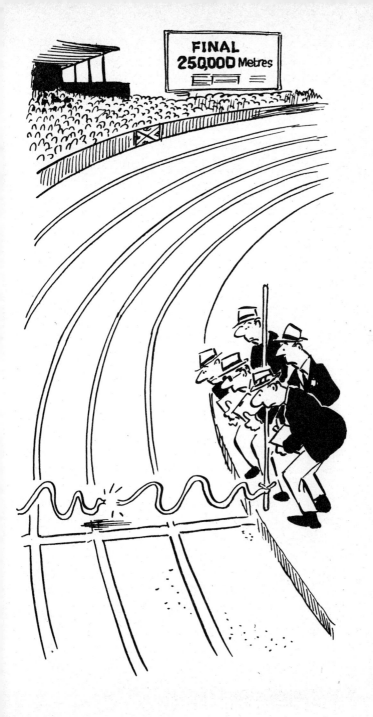

A study of Aberdeen school children showed that more boys than girls had crammed their feet into unsuitable shoes and were suffering from bunions.

A flourishing business in seventeenth-century Europe was importing the flesh of Egyptian mummies for use in medical treatment. When supplies ran short during epidemics, unscrupulous Alexandrians shipped the bodies of freshly-soused slaves.

Rhubarb and spinach are rich in oxalic acid, of which one-fifth of an ounce can be fatal.

The man with the longest penis in the Masters and Johnson study was just five feet seven inches tall.

In 1541 the Guild of English Surgeons resolved that 'no carpenter, smith, weaver or woman practise surgery'.

Paracelsus in the sixteenth century suggested that to make a homunculus – 'a true and living infant having all the members of a child that is born of a woman but much smaller' – you should warm some human semen and feed it with blood.

Fat American airmen at the USAF base at Lakenheath, Suffolk, were threatened with demotion if they failed to lose weight.

Children born feet-first were known as footlings, and were credited with the power of healing lumbago, back-ache, rheumatism and sprains by trampling on the sufferer with their gifted feet.

Americans swallow more than thirty million pounds weight of aspirin every year.

The odds against reaching your 100th birthday are about 12,500:1 if you are a man, but only 2,500:1 if you are a woman.

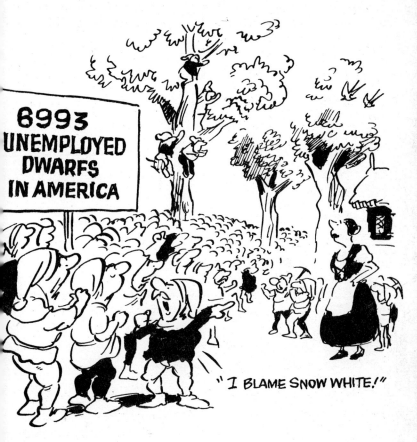

There are 7000 dwarfs in the United States.

A long-playing record of sounds from inside a mother's womb became a best-seller in Japan after it was shown to soothe crying babies. In tests, it stopped every one of 403 babies crying in an average 41 seconds, and put 161 of them completely to sleep. The record, a series of gentle thuds, is called 'Lullaby Inside Mum'.

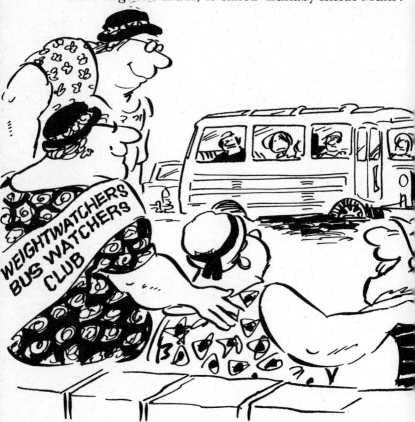

A bus carrying 28 members of the Wogga Wogga Weight-Watchers' Club sank up to its axles in a tarred car park.

A survey of coronary thrombosis in farmers revealed that those who did full-time physical work suffered 20 fatal heart attacks per 1000. Part-time physical workers had 61 per 1000; those who did no physical work had 116; and those who rented their farms out to others had 132. These last might care to know that, for the price of one new hospital, you can build at least 50 sports clubs.

The Peruvian camu-camu fruit contains 60 times more vitamin C than an orange.

More people commit suicide in summer than in winter, and in the afternoon than the morning.

Only one per cent of Frenchmen have enough energy left after the weekend to make love on Mondays.

HMS *Dido*'s arrival in Fiji in 1875 sparked off a measles epidemic that wiped out a quarter of the island's population in three months.

Road accidents in Britain kill more people than diphtheria, measles, plague, anthrax, dysentery, poliomyelitis, smallpox, whooping cough, tuberculosis and cholera combined.

Scotland might easily have escaped the Black Death were it not for greed. Hoping to take advantage of England's disease-weakened condition, a Scots army went marauding in 1349. The soldiers took back with them rather more than they had bargained for.

Eighty per cent of appendicitis cases occur before the age of 30.

More men than women in this country have lost ears through amputation or accident.

An old man congratulating himself on not having put on weight in middle age is likely only to have substituted youthful muscle for elderly fat.

One male doctor in 50 kills himself.

Tears can heal. They contain lysozyme, an antiseptic.

It is thought that a liking for the odour of oestrogen may account for the mosquitoes preference for women victims.

A man was treated in a Kuala Lumpur hospital for a sprained neck after a trained monkey, sent up a tree to gather coconuts, jumped on to his shoulders and began twisting his head.

Barnacles in the sea off Aberystwyth contained up to 20,000 parts per million of zinc – equivalent to a 14-stone man having three pounds of metal in his body.

Menstruating women in the Lele tribe are forbidden to cook or to poke their husbands' fires.

The heavy light-bulb wastage at Collin County Jail, Texas, was traced to 44-year-old prisoner Frank Reese, who had been eating them. The sheriff was invited to exhibit his man at the local TV station, where Reese duly obliged by taking a meal of 14 light-bulbs and the sheriff's sunglasses.

New Zealanders who drank more than two-and-a-half litres of cheap local sherry a week found their hair beginning to turn ginger. They also developed a brown skin colour, liver abnormality and anaemia.

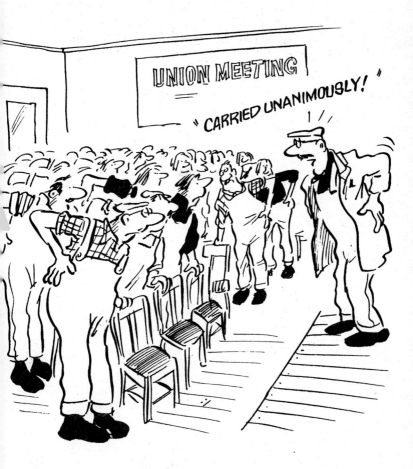

Thirteen million British working days are lost every year because of back-ache.

The coddled inhabitants of New York State have the highest ratio of doctors to patients in the USA.– 193 of them to every 100,000. The neglected folk of Nebraska have to get by with half that, but they have a life expectancy two-and-a-half years better than their over-doctored New York cousins.

Nerve impulses travel about 20 mph faster than the world helicopter speed record.

Subliminal attempts to persuade a cinema audience to buy refreshments by periodically flashing the word 'ice-cream' on to the screen for a fraction of a second, resulted only in a few complaints that the cinema was too cold.

John Bylsden, a bachelor of medicine at Oxford with 15 years' medical experience and four years of lecturing, was granted his doctor's degree in 1455 on the condition that he repaired the windows in the Hall of Congregation.

A bottle of milk left standing in daylight loses from a half to two-thirds of its riboflavin (vitamin B) within two hours.

Stuffy-nosed America spends 500 million dollars a year on cold cures.

Human eye-cells are sensitive enough to register light as dim as 100-billionth of a watt.

Penicillin allergy kills some 3000 people every year.

In 1971, a new weapon in the war against drug traffickers was unleashed in Marseilles – a Volkswagen camper with a roof-mounted snorkel and sniffing-gear for detecting the acetic anhydrides used to make heroin. When the sniffer's findings were analysed, it was found that it had put the finger on all the restaurants in the city, but no heroin labs. The machine had been responding to the smell of salad cream.

Researchers have discovered that Japanese people have longer large intestines than Europeans. Japanese women are accordingly flocking to private clinics to have 50 inches of intestine chopped out in an attempt to achieve the deathly Western skin-pallor so admired by beauty-conscious Orientals. A surgeon specialising in the operation said the extra length of intestine made the Japanese more susceptible to colon syndrome, which causes yellowing of the skin.

Nine holidaymakers were treated for donkey-bites at Bridlington in 1974.

Throwing excrement out of windows was banned in Paris by royal decree in 1372 and again in 1395.

An American searching for a calorie-free food tried powdered coal, glass and sand before settling for chopped surgical cotton and fruit juice.

A top hat could hold all the human ova to spawn the entire population of the world. To fertilise them would take a thimbleful of sperms.

The more drugs he prescribes, the more money a doctor in Japan makes.

Hark the herald angels sing
Beecham's Pills are just the thing.
For blessed peace and mercy mild
Two for mother, one for child

sang the congregation at a carol service in an impoverished East End parish. The vicar had been offered free hymn books by Beecham's, and had only allowed their use after what he thought was a thorough check for advertising matter.

The Hogben pregnancy test, which involves injecting concentrated urine into a female South African clawed toad, is positive if the toad spawns 50 to 200 eggs within 15 hours.

American doctors are paying up to $16,000 a year – more than the average British doctor's salary – to insure themselves against lawsuits from aggrieved patients.

A survey of 1300 motorists showed that the number of accidents rose in inverse proportion to the frequency of car-polishing. All-time non-polishers suffered an average of 198 accidents per 100; once-weekly polishers had only 76 per 100.

An American woman sold 30,000 oz of her milk for $3717 – about 60p a pint.

The Negritos of the Andaman Islands in the Bay of Bengal are ambidextrous but unable to wink.

Mediaeval law made it an offence to do anything which could reduce your own or anyone else's ability to serve king and country. Castration and the removal of front teeth were both strictly illegal.

Well-educated people get more colds than the unschooled, though the rich catch fewer than the poor.

A properly-conducted abortion is 12 times safer than having your tonsils out; a tonsillectomy is about as risky as taking contraception pills for 160 years.

If the number of doctors continues to increase at the present rate, within 500 years the entire population will be engaged in medical practice.

The study of medicine was not encouraged at Oxford during the middle ages. Merton College went so far as to ban it altogether.

When Lister's new hospital was opened in the last century the patients had to pay a deposit to cover the cost of burial should they not survive treatment.

When the US Army laboratories analysed four sacred Tibetan *pedung* pills, made from the Dalai Lama's stools, they found that the holy man had been eating wheat-flour 'of a coarse quality' and that he had no obstruction in his bile ducts.

Experiments on rats suggest that the human lifespan could be extended by a fifth if we ate three or four times as much vitamin A. Other authorities say the average adult's daily need is satisfied by one peach, a tablespoon of cooked carrot, 50 sprigs of parsley, two red peppers, a tablespoon of dandelion greens or two cans of sardines.

The kernels of plums, apricots, cherries and apple pips can all produce cyanide poisoning.

The Maudsley Hospital has found that about 8 per cent of the people it treats for chronic alcoholism kill themselves within five years.

Following the discovery of a link between cigarette-smoking and lung cancer, American tobacco-growers retorted with a campaign to demonstrate that 95 per cent of the victims of fatal air-crashes in the previous year had eaten pickles.

A company in New York called Pregnancy Without Fear developed and marketed an egg-shaped satin pillow, pleasantly adorned with lace and coloured rosettes. If you stuck it up your jumper you looked six months pregnant. 'All the joys of pregnancy without pain . . .' and no trouble getting a seat on the bus.

Blindness is so common in some African villages that ropes are put up to guide women to the wells.

Four tons of rotten teeth are pulled from children in England and Wales every year.

Fat schoolchildren usually eat less than their slim playmates.

Thirty-eight Haitian refugees were picked up, half-starved and semi-conscious after nine days in an open boat. When asked why they were all blindfolded, they replied: 'We did not wish to witness each other's destruction'.

Ambroise Paré, a sixteenth-century French surgeon, was accused of being a crank when he refused to prescribe crushed Egyptian mummy to a patient injured in an accident.

Claude Bernard was disconcerted to find that the best-selling medicine at the pharmacy where he worked seemed to vary in composition from day to day. He later discovered it was a random mixture of any left-over or spoiled drugs that happened to be around.

A London dentist of the 1770s, Martin von Butchall, was famous not so much for his skill in his chosen profession but for the embalmed body of his first wife which he kept on display in his home. His second wife, however, objected to her constant presence, so the body was presented to the Royal College of Surgeons, where it was kept until 1941.

Surgeons opening the abdomen of a three-month-old Syrian girl, thought to have a tumour, found three developing foetuses inside.

The bacteria living in and on a human body would fill a teacup.

Queen Amelia of Portugal had X-ray pictures taken of ladies at court to demonstrate the evils of wearing over-tight corsets.

Your hair standing on end when you are frightened is the remains of a reaction designed to frighten away the enemy by making you look taller.

Leaving aside dwarfs and giants, virtually the whole world population can be included within a two-foot span in height. Only a negligible number are shorter than 4 ft 7 in or taller than 6 ft 7 in – which makes the tallest less than half again as high as the shortest. No such rule applies to weight, however, A normal man can often be twice the weight of a normal girl.

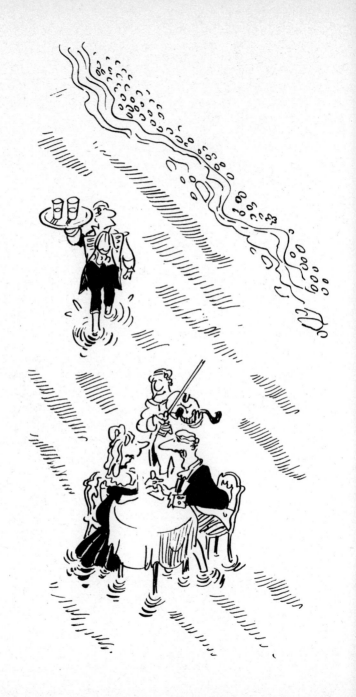

No one went into the sea before 1750 unless they wanted to cure the bite of a mad dog. After that year the medical profession began to wake up to the potential of seawater as an aid to general health. But you had to drink it, not go for a swim.

Those born in January, February and March are more likely to suffer from schizophrenia and manic depression than those born later in the year.

When X-rays were first invented some people thought them indecent, and Londoners could buy 'X-ray-proof' underclothes.

Bald men should beware of cheap wigs. The Hair Extension Centre has warned that metal partitions in centrally heated offices generate static electricity and can deal a nasty shock to anyone brushing against them wearing a 'cheap hairpiece'.

Cyclamate sweeteners, banned after a furore in Britain and the USA, have never been shown to have killed a single human being. To consume the equivalent of the amount that produced cancer in rats, you would have to drink several hundred glasses of cyclamate-sweetened drink every day. Sugar, however, is a contributory factor in several serious complaints.

To cure dropsy: chop off the patient's head, turn him upside down to allow the offending liquids to drain away, replace the head and a complete recovery will follow – or so traditional Greek medicine assures us.

Some 'insomniacs' believe they have not slept only because they have spent most of the night dreaming they are awake.

A Hungarian scientist found that mice housed within magnetic fields looked younger and were 30 per cent more active than ordinary mice. They also acquired total immunity from cancer metastases.

The first recorded cases in Britain of botulism (poisoning from canned or sausage meat) were a party of eight who died in Scotland in 1922 after eating potted duck.

An Australian company has perfected a slide fastener for zipping surgical incisions together instead of stitching them.

Women are more liable to chilblains than men.

The Russian surgeon Voronoff was invited by Encyclopaedia Britannica to contribute the entry on Rejuvenation. He wrote: 'The only remedy for ageing is to graft a young testicle, whether that of a young human being or of an ape.' His essay was published in only one edition of the learned work, and has not appeared since. True to his principles, though, 160 times between 1920 and 1951 Voronoff transplanted chimpanzees' testicles into elderly men.

French aristocrats had a passion for enemas. Louis XIII had 212, together with 215 purges and 47 bleedings in one year. In Louis XIV's reign an enema a day was commonplace, the Canon of Troyes managing 2,190 in two years. A machine consisting of a stool with a manually retractable pin was sold for self-administration, and even pet dogs had to undergo the treatment.

Half of all admissions to medical wards of women aged 15 to 40 result from self-poisoning.

An Irish cure for mumps was to lead the sufferer on reins three times round a pigsty.

In the Middle Ages it was believed that women's ears were erogenous zones and should be kept appropriately covered.

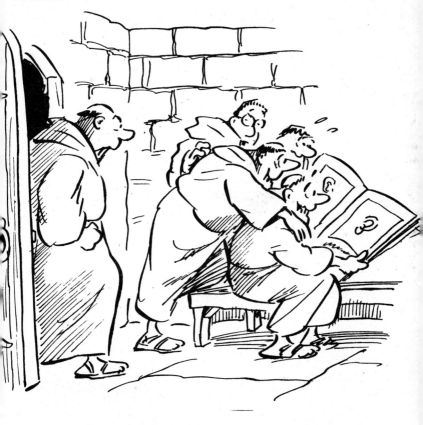

Analysis of Beecham's Pills in 1912 revealed that they contained aloes, ginger and soap. With production costs at ½d, they sold for 2s 9d, a 6000 per cent mark-up.

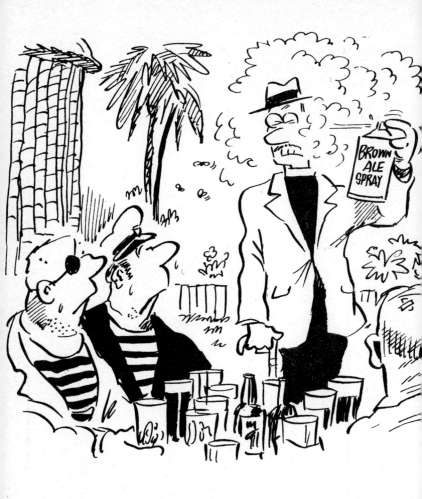

Mosquitoes do not like beer, according to Vienna dermatologist Professor Anton Luger. He advised outdoor topers to sink enough ale to promote a mild (or bitter) perspiration. The small amount of beer in the sweat is enough to drive a thirsty insect spiralling off in search of a Baptist minister.

The only legal source of bodies for dissection in the last century was the gallows, and a thriving black market dealt in bodies snatched from new graves or even from hospitals by fake relatives. When the asking price rose from 2 gns to around 15 gns some doctors formed an Anatomy Club to resist the tide of inflation. The move was unsuccessful and one of the doctors, Joshua Brookes, found his initiative rewarded with decomposing bodies dumped on his doorstep.

Drug companies send the average GP his own weight in advertising material every year.

Isabeau of Bavaria, Queen of France at the end of the fourth century, enriched her complexion with a lotion of boar's brains, wolf's blood and crocodile glands.

Veins have valves to stop the blood rushing to your feet when you stand up.

The largest gland in the body is the liver, weighing between three and three-and-a-half pounds.

The original Siamese twins, Chang and Eng (Left and Right in Thai) are called the Chinese twins in Siam as their parents came from China.

In the eighteenth century a physician was recognised by his golden-headed cane. The handle concealed a pomander for combatting the odours of patients' homes and persons.

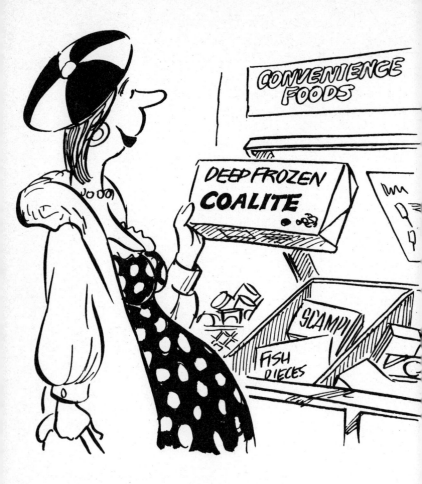

A list compiled by the BBC of pregnant women's cravings included 261 for fruit, 105 for vegetables, 107 for special foods such as pickles, 35 for coal, 17 for soap, 15 for disinfectant and 14 for toothpaste.

In 1900 a new-born American baby had less chance of surviving a week than a man of 90.

The creed of the Gender Identity Clinic in Baltimore, one of six clinics set up in the US to perform sex-change operations, is 'If the mind cannot be changed to fit the body, we should consider changing the body to fit the mind'. Altogether more than 1000 such operations have been performed worldwide.

A corpse hanging on the gallows minus his hands or feet usually meant a barren woman lived nearby. Contact with a dead criminal was thought to induce fertility.

Every time you smoke a cigarette you use up 20 to 30 milligrams of vitamin C.

Phenothiazines, drugs commonly used to treat schizophrenia, were first used as insecticides and to banish worms in pet animals.

Members of the Hi-Lo Tops, an Oregon slimming club, who show a gain in weight at the weekly check, have to stand a large statue of a pig in their front garden.

Fresh, healthy urine is virtually free from bacteria while saliva spat from the mouth contains up to 1000 million microbes per cubic centimetre.

The earliest medical thermometers, which were extremely large, contained so much mercury that it took at least five minutes to register a temperature.

A 40-year-old married man admitted to hospital for a routine hernia operation in 1963 was found to be the owner of a rudimentary uterus and one Fallopian tube.

99

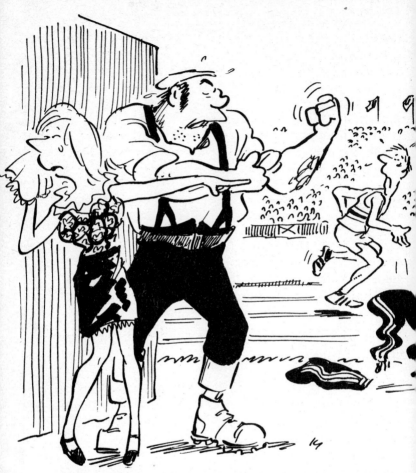

Dr Craig Sharp, medical adviser to Britain's Olympic canoeists, has said that, contrary to popular belief, sexual activity can improve *athletic performance. One Olympic middle-distance champion broke the world record an hour after intercourse, and a British athlete ran a four-minute mile only one-and-a-half hours after coming to grips.*

100

At the beginning of this century the Governor of the Phillipines gave an American doctor permission to infect two groups of prisoners with bubonic plague and beri-beri. The lucky men received tobacco as payment.

In the twelfth century the growth of the various parts of the foetus was believed to be regulated by the planets: the brain formed under Mercury and the liver under Jupiter.

Taking sleeping tablets reduces the amount of time spent dreaming.

Andrew Still, founder of American osteopathy, claimed that with bone manipulation he had caused three inches of hair to grow on a bald head. His textbook, published when he was 82, explained how manipulation could cure everything from dandruff to yellow fever and maintained that germs do not exist.

Before the advent of silicone, breasts were enlarged with implants of ivory.

The centrepiece of James Graham's Temple of Health, which opened in London in 1780, was his Celestial Bed. It was 12 ft long by 9 ft wide, supported by 40 pillars and topped with a dome containing 'balmy and ethereal spices' and lined with mirrors. The therapeutic force of the bed was provided by 15 cwt of magnets and a squadron of 'vestal virgins' including the future Lady Hamilton, Nelson's mistress.

Hundreds of people taken to hospital in Morocco suffering from food poisoning were found to have eaten food in which aircraft-engine oil had been substituted for olive oil.

101

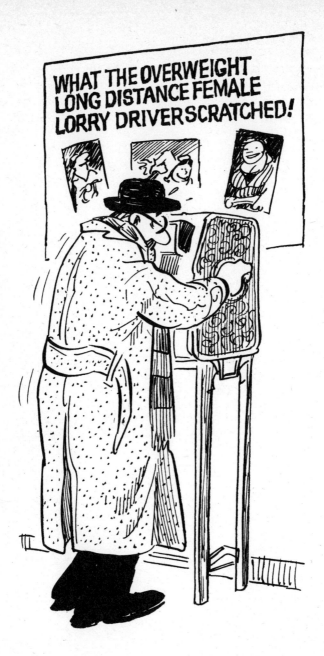

Three-quarters of the population now suffer from an itch they cannot publicly scratch, pruritis ani. *Itchy-bottom-ologists say it strikes hardest at overweight women long-distance lorry drivers on the Pill who wear too-tight trousers and spend too much time on plastic seats.*

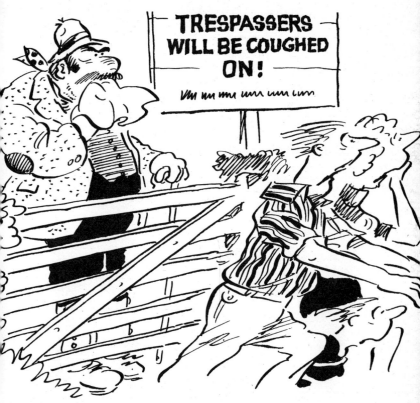

Aside from the familiar housemaid's knee and tennis elbow, the range of occupational diseases includes potter's asthma, farmer's lung, wool-sorter's disease, chimney-sweep's cancer and grinder's rot.

Fat people are more likely than slim ones to suffer from rheumatoid and osteo-arthritis, diabetes, gall-bladder disease, high blood pressure, infertility, varicose veins, toxaemia of pregnancy, coronary thrombosis, hiatus hernia, obstetric complications, cirrhosis of the liver and cerebral thrombosis. However, they are less likely to suffer from tuberculosis or to kill themselves. Half the British population is overweight.

The daily heat output of the average man would boil 30 litres of freezing water.

When the Thames shrank to a trickle during June 1858, the month of the Great Stink, MPs protected themselves from stench and disease by having boat-loads of lime dumped on the Palace of Westminster's terraces, and sheets of canvas fixed over the windows and coated with zinc chloride.

A 19-year-old Sardinian student was reported satisfactory after a four-hour surgical exploration of his stomach had yielded two coins, some keys, two fish-forks and 38 coffee-spoons.

It has been estimated that drug companies spend more on advertising than on research into new drugs.

In Ancient Egypt there were medical consultants for baldness and premature greying, and a Specialist on the Royal Anus.

The use of hypnotism as a stage entertainment was outlawed in Britain in 1952.

Christien Heineken, a child prodigy, knew the whole of the Bible at fourteen months; at two and a half he could read German and Latin and speak them fluently; at three he could add, subtract and multiply; in his fourth year he learned 220 songs, 80 psalms and 1500 Latin verses. He died aged four years and four months.

Fifty-eight per cent of all Americans suffer from obesity.

King James I was so fond of a day's hunting that he would not leave his saddle even to relieve himself.

Jerome Irving Wardale, who died leaving a nine-million dollar empire founded on natural medicine magazines, blamed most of the world's ills on sugar. Hitler, he said, was an obvious sugar addict. And was it merely coincidence that the Boston Strangler liked sugar? Or that the FBI found an empty Coca-Cola bottle in the Dallas book depository from which Lee Harvey Oswald was supposed to have shot John Kennedy?

There are 520 muscles in the body, and none has a name longer than the *levator labii superioris aloequae nasi.*

The body has a number of resonant frequencies. At five cycles per second, for instance, the shoulder-blades will heave painfully, and a sound of 20 cycles will literally rock the eyeballs in their sockets. Other low frequencies have caused embarrassment in recording studios by provoking such reactions as contraction of the throat and involuntary defaecation.

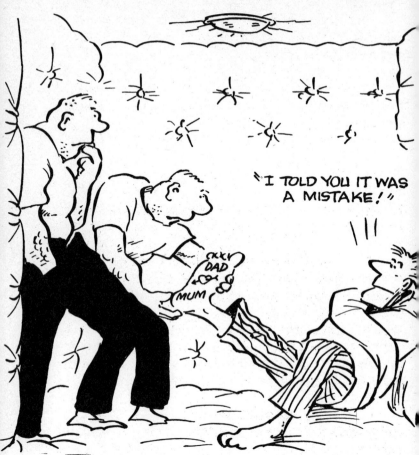

A tattooed man is more likely to go to jail than one without tattoos, but less likely to go to a mental hospital.

To help cure the ills of 1890s America, the first exponents of chiropractics – spine manipulation – invented the 'electroencephaloneuromentimpograph'.

In most clinical trials, nearly a third of the patients given placebos of powdered chalk claim some improvement in their condition.

An early anaesthetic was the 'soporific sponge'. Soaked in opium, mandragora, ground ivy, lettuce juice and hemlock and allowed to dry, it was moistened before an operation and pushed up the patient's nose.

Ancient Greeks believed that if a woman remained childless for too long, the angry womb (*hysteros*) began to wander round the body causing havoc – or 'hysteria'.

People who 'can't sleep' average only three-quarters of an hour less each night than good sleepers.

The ten habits most likely to hasten you to an early grave, listed in 1922 by Czech doctor Arnold Lorand, were alcohol, over-eating, tobacco, sexual in-discretion, uncleanliness, ambition, avarice, anger, vanity and avoidance of parenthood. Arsenic, he said, was rejuvenating.

In 1970 British doctors wrote 44 million prescriptions for sedatives, anti-depressants and tran-quillisers, 30 million for antibiotics, 17.6 million for cough mixtures, and 3.4 million for laxatives, purgatives and suppositories.

Two hundred thousand frowns add up to one wrinkle.

The average height of the Watusi is 6 ft 5 in.

Average life-expectancy in Britain was 18 in the Iron Age, 22 in the first century BC, 33 in the Middle Ages, 33.5 in the period 1687-91, 35.5 in 1789, 40.9 in 1836-54, 49.2 in 1900-02, and 66.8 in 1947. Current figures are 68.1 years for men, and 74.0 for women.

Umbilical cords can be anything from seven inches to four feet long. An active foetus literally ties the cord in knots.

Britain loses 100 times more working days through sickness than through strikes.

In the last century, alcohol was the most popular medicine for insanity. Mental hospitals spent more on beer, wines and spirits than on all other drugs put together.

In Britain the odds against having twins are 90 to 1, in Belgium 56 to 1, in South America 125 to 1, and in one Nigerian tribe 22 to 1.

To discover what happened to the food he ate, Spallanzani, an eighteenth-century Italian investigator, carved wooden tubes with holes cut in the sides. He put pieces of meat into the holes, put the tubes into his mouth, closed his eyes and swallowed. After the contraption had been in place for a while, he would poke a finger into his throat, throw the whole lot up again, and examine the meat to see how it had changed.

The brain of the Russian novelist Ivan Turgenev was exactly twice as big as that of the French writer Anatole France.

108

One apothecary in the early days of St Bartholemew's Hospital, London, applied time and motion principles to dispensing. Having gathered his crowd of patients, he formed them into groups by ailment – cough, stomach ache, etc., and each group would stand in turn to receive its common medication.

Fifty years ago the most common cause of insanity among educated Americans was brain syphilis.

Young men think about sex once every 15 minutes.

It was really smallpox and not Cortez who conquered Mexico for Spain. It killed half the Aztec population in six months.

Women have been known to remain pregnant for 13 or 14 months. The babies are believed to lie dormant in the womb.

Somebody attempts suicide in the USA every minute.

Non-identical twins can have different fathers.

To cure a courtly lady who had lost the use of her arms, Avicenna, a tenth-century Arab physician, stripped off her veil, which made her blush, then stooped down and hoisted her skirt over her head. The woman hastily pulled it down again, and realised she could use her arms after all. Avicenna attributed the cure to the blush which, he said, 'dissolved the erring humours'.

An outbreak of poisoning in Holland in 1960 was traced to a 'new, improved' margarine containing an additive to prevent it spitting in the frying pan.

Lorry-driver Pantaleo Terranova was in bed with his wife one stormy night while Italian electricity board employees tried to repair a cable on the roof. They broke some tiles and a deluge of icy water drenched the couple. Pantaleo sued the board for £100,000 damages to compensate him for the resulting 66 days of impotence and public scorn. After four years of legal bickering, he was awarded £300.

Pure liquid nicotine is highly poisonous. A 40 milligrams dose, roughly the contents of two cigarettes, is usually fatal.

Mrs Rita Castro of Texas gave birth to a boy on 9 December, 1966. His twin sister was born 30 days later.

A *Sunday Pictorial* request for information about virgin births produced 19 claimants who believed their child had no father. One could not be disproved.

Bloodletting was supposed to clear the mind, improve the memory, clean the stomach, warm the marrow, improve hearing, halt tears, feed and cleanse the blood and bring long life. It was not recommended for the aged.

Marie Antoinette and Jayne Mansfield had identical bust-measurements.

A popular old remedy for whooping cough was a spoonful of woodlice, bruised and mixed with breast-milk.

The urge to take 40 winks after a large meal is caused by chemicals in the food itself. A steak alone contains enough tryptophane (converted by the body to serotin, the 'sleep juice') to make you feel drowsy.

Malaria was originally thought to be caused by the unwholesome atmosphere in which it thrived. Hence the name *mal aria*, bad air.

A sudden six per cent increase in the Japanese birth rate occurred in 1965 because 1966 was the Year of the Fire Horse. Any girl born in that year was supposed to be so domineering that no man in his right mind would marry her.

Our hands have up to 1300 nerve endings per square inch.

Orthopaedic surgeon Brian Reeves of Leeds has invented a boot with springs in its heel for patients with broken feet or legs.

An American woman weighing 33 st. went on a liquid diet and became pregnant when her weight was just under 22 st. During pregnancy, at the end of which she produced a normal child, she lost another 8 st.

A woman in Herne Hill, London woke up one morning to find the dead body of a man wedged in her bedroom window. Police deduced that he was a burglar who had died from a heart attack.

Women have smaller hearts than men in relation to body-size, and smaller lungs.

So many people died of the Black Death in southern France that the Pope formally consecrated the River Rhone at Avignon. Corpses thrown into the water might therefore be considered to have had a Christian burial.

The oldest doctors' book of rules in existence, the 4000-year-old Babylonian Code of Hammurabi, ordered: 'If a physician shall make a severe wound . . . on the slave of a free man and kill him, he shall replace the slave with another.

The brain's nerve cells use up one-fifth of our oxygen intake.

The blood of a 20-a-day smoker contains twice as much carbon monoxide as that of a traffic policeman.

A perceptible deterioration in the quality of the bread made by a Paris baker was remarked on after sanitary inspectors closed down a connection between the reservoir from which the bakery drew its water and the lavatories of neighbouring houses.

A Rumanian doctor has claimed to rejuvenate patients with a drug similar to one used as a dental anaesthetic.

Up to 1940 there were 122 recorded cases of babies crying while still inside the womb.

Mediaeval surgeons consulted the stars before operating. If the moon was in Taurus they avoided the neck and throat, if in Aquarius the legs, and if in Pisces the feet were safe from the knife.

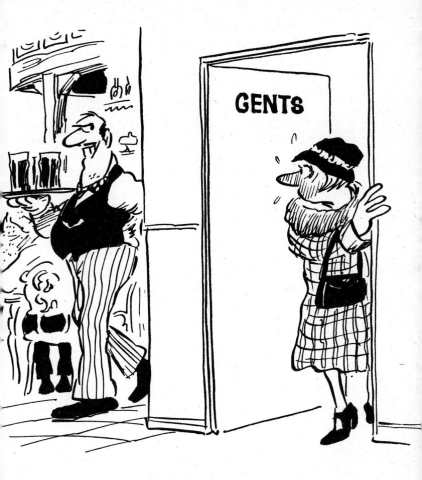

The Permissive Age has so far left intact a profitable sideline for some pub landlords. They leave empty contraceptive machines in their lavatories and rely on customers being too embarrassed to demand their money back.

You are more likely to die from a lightning strike in England than from the bite of an adder.

Children conceived on the day of ovulation have a 57:43 chance of being girls. A child conceived six or more days beforehand has a 70 per cent chance of being a boy.

One person in 20 has an extra rib.

Mrs Sarah Mapp, an eighteenth-century London bone-setter, was scorned by the medical profession but had her revenge when one doctor sent her a hoax patient. She dislocated his shoulder with the instruction that he should return a month later if the doctor could not fix it.

A London hospital studied adult males who had suffered from mumps. They were able to report that the common fear that mumps cause sterility is groundless.

Blood collections in North Wales during the Second World War showed that proportionally fewer people with English surnames belonged to blood groups O and B than those with names such as Jones, Williams and Morgan.

Before the advent of North Sea gas, parents cured children of whooping cough by marching them round the local gasworks.

In a New York survey, one-third of the men claiming to have been circumcised were mistaken. And so were one-third of those claiming to be intact.

It used to be believed that the bite of a mad dog could be cured by swiftly applying a 'hair of the dog'.

114

A 22 st. 7 lb Los Angeles woman lost 9 st. in 117 days by fasting.

Not only insomniacs wake during the night. Most adults wake four or five times, but so briefly that they do not remember.

Bad news for Turkish bath enthusiasts. There is less water content in fat than in any other bodily tissue – even bone.

When the rage for psychoanalysis was at its peak shortly after the Second World War, American parents regularly took two-year-old children to be analysed.

All spiders are poisonous. The 'harmless' ones are simply too weak to bite through human skin.

The heart of a 90-year-old pumps only half as much at a time as it did when its owner was 20.

An American company, Smell It Like It Is Inc., sells T-shirts impregnated with perfumes which are activated by body-heat. Among the 200 smells on offer are banana, pine, orange, beer, cold lamb and Kentucky fried chicken.

A mediaeval doctor was expected to have many talents. The king's favourites would be sent on diplomatic missions or personal royal errands. One was entrusted with building a royal residence near Nottingham.

Blood is pumped through the aorta, the main artery, at such pressure that, if it were opened, it would spout 6 ft into the air.

A comet which appeared in 676 heralded an outbreak of pestilence in Barking.

If their patients died, surgeons in Ancient Egypt had their hands cut off.

The liver can clean one-quarter oz alcohol from the bloodstream every hour, which is good news for the man who wants to spend the rest of his life drinking half a tot of whisky or half a pint of beer an hour. He will never get drunk.

Laid end to end, the tiny tubes from your liver would stretch from London to Brighton.

A blonde Venezuelan stripper who performs nightly at a club in Caracas writes to her mother every week enclosing a doctor's certificate to show she is still a virgin.

Spirits of wine, later known as brandy, was introduced to medicine around 1300 by the French physician Arnauld de Villeneuve. No doubt intoxicated by his discovery, he dubbed it 'water of immortality'.

When heroin was first isolated in Germany in 1898 it was heralded as a great cure for opium addiction.

A baby boom devastated British maternity wards in the late summer of 1974 – nine months after Government-imposed power-restrictions had compelled an early-evening television black-out. The only exception was a small part of Yorkshire where, apparently, they had thought of something better to do.

In the Middle Ages it was usual for a doctor to demand his fee before treatment to avoid the patient either dying before paying or haggling over the cost once he had recovered.

Each cubic millimetre of blood contains 5 million red cells. Your body contains 10 pints of blood.

During surgery hours in 1970, the average British GP wrote one prescription every six minutes.

Spartans were figure-conscious. Any young men showing signs of overweight at monthly naked line-ups had to do special exercises.

Red blood cells live for 100 days, white for 13 days.

Cato insisted that the citizens of Rome had no need of doctors but should use his remedies – cabbages and herbs. He allowed two exceptions: fractures could be healed with a magic song and dislocations by chanting '*Huat, hanat, ista, sista, domiabo, damnaistra*'. He was predeceased by his two main patients, his wife and son.

One in five women in Lancashire believe cancer is infectious, hereditary or a punishment for youthful sin.

A group of schoolboys nominated a leading dermatologist 'sportsman of the year' for having written that 'skin diseases in civilised countries due to excessive washing are commoner than those attributed to dirt'.

117

A child with one fat parent has a 40 to 50 per cent chance of being fat, too. If both parents are overweight, he has an 80 per cent chance.

Though Harvey is generally credited with the discovery of the circulation of the blood in 1616, the Chinese Emperor Hwang-Ti wrote in 2650 BC that 'All the blood in the body is under the control of the heart. The blood flows continuously in a circle and never stops'.

Poisonous snakes kill 40,000 people a year.

The US Department of Health, Education and Welfare has pronounced that there is enough evidence to make palm-reading worth researching as an aid to diagnosis.

Drug tolerance varies dramatically. In tests on one sleep-inducing compound, some people felt drowsy after only 75 milligrams, others felt alert after doses nearly 15 times greater.

Reporting that the number of Frenchmen with below-average sperm counts has risen from 29 to 71 per cent, a doctor blamed insomnia, overwork, depression, anxiety and the use of tranquillisers.

It used to be thought that noise conquered disease. A dentist suggested that the cholera raging through London in 1832 should be checked by surrounding the city with cannons firing every hour.

You will very likely be poisoned if you eat balloon fish in Japan. The same fish is completely harmless when caught off the coast of West Africa.

Hippocrates treated cerebral haemorrhage by putting myrrh and sulphur up the patient's nose to make him sneeze.

Infibulation, an operation in which the foreskin is pulled over the end of the penis and secured by a ring passed through two specially-pierced holes, was a popular way of preventing adolescents from masturbating in ancient Greece and Rome. A nineteenth-century German professor of medicine held that the practice should be revived to stop impecunious bachelors from breeding.

Two women in Russia and one in the United States can distinguish colours with their fingertips.

When Knud Kjer Jensen tried to stand up after falling into a Danish barberry thicket, he fainted and fell over again, his whole body bristling with inch-long thorns. So far doctors have managed to remove 23,982 of them.

A recent survey found that only one person in three considered himself to be in good health. Of these fortunate few 95 per cent complained of some ailment within the preceding two weeks.

More male babies than female are born to mothers of blood group AB, fathers who have been exposed to radiation, and members of the United States Air Force.

Oriental monks took hashish to subdue their sexual passions and help themselves remain celibate.